DON'T DIE ALONE

Quarto

This edition published in 2026 by Chartwell Books,
an imprint of The Quarto Group
142 West 36th Street, 4th Floor
New York, NY 10018 USA
T (212) 779-4972
www.Quarto.com

Contains content originally published as *The Loneliness Problem*, 2024, by Chartwell Books.

10 9 8 7 6 5 4 3 2 1

ISBN: 978-0-7858-4904-9

Publisher: Wendy Friedman
Publishing Director: Meredith Mennitt
Editor: Cathy Davis
Designer: Kate Sinclair
Cover Designer: Angelika Piwowarczyk
All stock design elements ©Shutterstock

Printed in Malaysia, PC1025

This book provides general information. It should not be relied upon as recommending or promoting any specific diagnosis or method of treatment for a particular condition. It is not intended as a substitute for medical advice or for direct diagnosis and treatment of a medical or psychological condition by a qualified physician or therapist. Readers who have questions about a particular condition, possible treatments for that condition, or possible reactions from the condition or its treatment should consult a physician, therapist, or other qualified healthcare professional.

EEA Representation, WTS Tax d.o.o.,
Žanova ulica 3, 4000 Kranj, Slovenia.
www.wts-tax.si

DON'T DIE ALONE

chartwell
books

CONTENTS

INTRODUCTION

Many view loneliness as a state of solitude or being alone, but one can be alone and not feel lonely. Thus, neuroscience researcher John Cacioppo, who has studied loneliness for more than twenty years, defines loneliness as "*perceived* social isolation," which we experience when we feel disconnected from others. Loneliness, he says, is a state of mind in which people may feel empty, alone, and unwanted, feelings that arise when a lack of social connection persists over a long period of time, usually accompanied by a lack of deep personal connection with trusted friends or family.

Loneliness is often associated with social isolation, poor social skills, introversion, and depression. People who are lonely crave human contact often, but their depressed state of mind makes it more difficult to form social connections. People who lack confidence in themselves often believe that they are unworthy of the attention or regard of other people, which can lead to increased isolation and chronic loneliness.

According to Cacioppo, our brains respond to the feeling of being on the outside by going into self-preservation mode. In that mode, our brains ramp up the stories we tell ourselves about what's happening (*I'm not likable; they think I'm weird*), creating stories that often are not true (*other people just don't like me; I don't have anything in common with them*) or exaggerate our worst fears and insecurities (*I'll never belong; I'll always be alone; I'm not lovable*). When we feel lonely, what we most need to do is seek connection. When we fail to do so, loneliness multiplies by keeping us afraid to reach out.

Loneliness can also result from our modern lifestyles, which are not only fast-paced but increasingly lack the kinds of tight-knit communities or churches that long sustain people. Now, thanks to the availability of the internet and social media, it's also possible for us to get whatever we want or need from the "safety" of our own homes. We may believe we're connecting on social media, but long-term, ongoing, face-to-face, and one-on-one interactions are needed to alleviate loneliness.

If, like many, you are feeling lonelier these days or feeling more disconnected than truly, deeply connected to others, this book is designed to help you develop the kind of interpersonal skills that will help you expand your social network, deepen your relationships, avoid the kind of soul-crushing loneliness that can be devastating, and live a more fulfilling life.

Let's begin by discussing the depth of the loneliness problem.

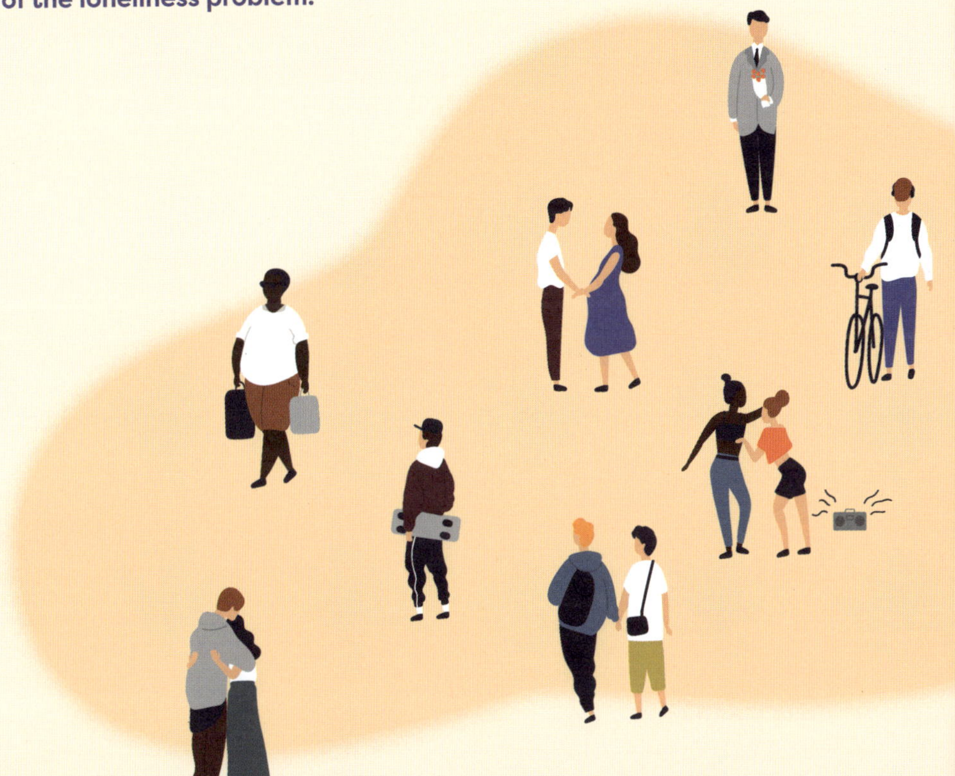

"I have spent whole decades inside and alone, whether or not there were any people around."

LIDIA YUKNAVITCH

CHAPTER 1

OUR NATIONAL LONELINESS

THE GROWING ENDEMIC

Many recent studies have confirmed that our loneliness problem is endemic and growing in America. *Even pre-COVID*, around 50 percent of American adults reported feeling lonely. That seems startling enough, but these facts may also surprise you:

Our young adults are lonely.

Some of the highest rates of loneliness occur in young adults, and it has increased every year between 1976 and 2019. While the highest rates of social isolation are found among older adults, young adults are almost *twice as likely* to report feeling lonely than those over sixty-five. Addiction to phones and social media is a factor.

We have fewer friends.

Ninety percent of people who aren't lonely or socially isolated reported having three or more confidants, while 49 percent of Americans in 2021 reported having *three or fewer close friends*, almost double the 27 percent who reported the same in 1990.

We feel disconnected.

A 2022 study found that when people were asked how close they felt to others, only 39 percent of American adults reported feeling very emotionally connected to others.

More of us live alone.

In 1960, single-person households accounted for only 13 percent of all US households, while in 2022, that number more than doubled to 29 percent of all households.

We don't see it as a major problem.

Despite such a high prevalence of loneliness and social isolation, less than 20 percent of individuals who reported often or always feeling lonely or isolated recognized it as a major problem.

IT'S DETRIMENTAL TO YOUR HEALTH

According to Dr. Vivek H. Murthy, Surgeon General of the United States, loneliness is associated with a greater risk of cardiovascular disease, dementia, stroke, depression, anxiety, and premature death. The mortality impact of being socially disconnected is similar to that caused by smoking up to fifteen cigarettes a day. It is even greater than that associated with obesity and physical inactivity. Healthy people who are more socially connected live longer, while those who experience social deficits, including isolation, loneliness, and poor-quality relationships (regardless of age, health status, socioeconomic status, and health practices) are more likely to die earlier, regardless of the cause.

Loneliness and social isolation also cause a lack of social connection in our schools, workplaces, and civic organizations, thereby diminishing performance, productivity, and engagement. A lack of social connection influences an individual's educational attainment, workplace satisfaction, economic prosperity, and overall feelings of well-being and life fulfillment. These negative effects can be so devastating our government created the National Strategy to Advance Social Connection.

LONELY PEOPLE DIE EARLY

In a meta-analysis of studies on loneliness, researchers found that living with air pollution increases your odds of dying early by 5 percent, living with obesity by 20 percent, excessive drinking by 30 percent, and loneliness by a whopping 45 percent.

CONNECTION IS A BASIC HUMAN NEED

Social connection is a basic human need, as essential to survival as food, water, and shelter. Humans have always relied on others to help them meet their basic needs, so much so that our brains were wired to foster social connections. In ancient times, the necessity for food gathering and protection from wild animals meant that people truly needed each other for survival. While we may be able to endure long periods without social connection today, living in isolation or outside the group means having to fulfill the many difficult demands of survival on one's own. Despite current advancements—the internet food delivery, automation, remote entertainment— that now allow us to fulfill many of our needs without leaving home, doing so requires far more effort, and the isolation that results reduces one's chances of living a fulfilling life. Despite advancements, our biological need to connect remains.

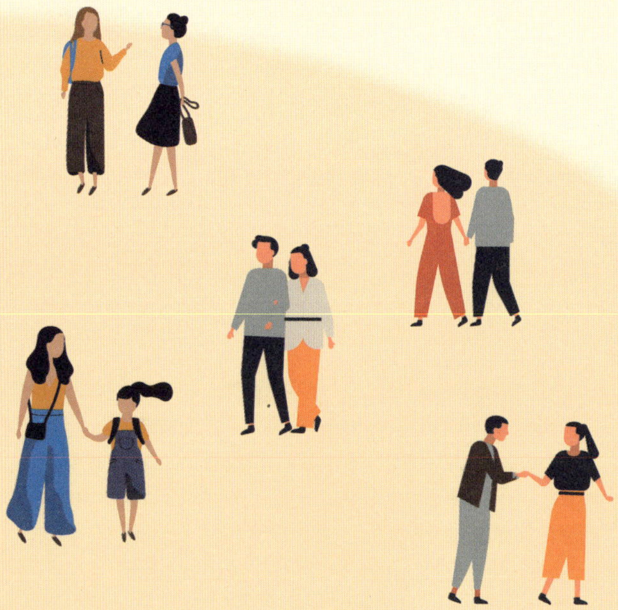

"To grow into adulthood as a social species is not to become autonomous and solitary. It's to become one on whom others can depend. Our brains and our biology have been shaped to favor this outcome. It's why connection matters."

JOHN CACIOPPO,

NEUROSCIENTIST

THE THREE ASPECTS OF SOCIAL CONNECTION

Social connection can encompass the interactions, relationships, roles, and sense of connection individuals, communities, or society may experience. Your level of social connection is not determined simply by the number of close relationships you have but in these three ways:

STRUCTURAL

The number of relationships, variety of relationships (coworkers, friends, family, neighbors), and frequency of interactions you have with others. Household size, friend circle size, and marital/partner status affect your structural connection.

How would you rate your life in terms of structural relationships? Do you have enough variety? Where do you need to find more friends?

FUNCTIONAL

The degree to which you can rely on others for various needs, such as emotional support, mentorship, or help in a crisis.

Do you have enough functional relationships? Who provides emotional support on a regular basis? List five people to whom you feel close enough to call upon them when you need them.

QUALITATIVE

The degree to which relationships and interactions with others are positive, helpful, or satisfying versus negative, unhelpful, or unsatisfying. This indicates your level of relationship satisfaction, relationship strain, social inclusion, or exclusion.

How's the quality of your social connections? How many close friends do you have, ones with whom you share the most intimate details of your life?

Which quality relationships would you like to deepen further?

Do you have dysfunctional relationships that you'd like to improve? Which ones can you address and work to improve?

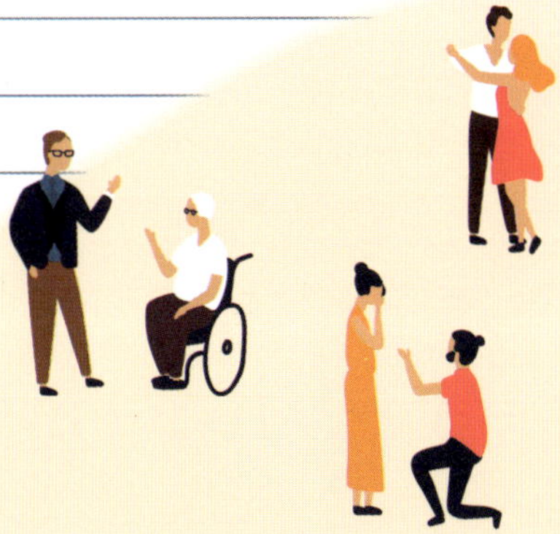

WHO'S IN YOUR CIRCLES?

According to British evolutionary psychologist Dr. Robin Dunbar, we have "circles of friendships." If you place yourself in the center of the circle, the inner circle is your qualitative or intimate friendships with whom you share the deepest bonds of mutual affection and trust. These are romantic partners, family, and close friends, our strongest emotional bonds, who provide ongoing protection, support, and emotional sustenance. The middle circle would be your functional friendships, people who offer shared support and connection, primarily on a reciprocal basis. We don't rely on them, but we know they would step up if needed. The outer circle would be structural friends, members of a larger community, neighbors, colleagues, classmates, and acquaintances who help you feel part of a collective. Dr. Dunbar says that we allocate 60 percent of our time and energy to our inner circle, typically less than five people. He warns that relationships with these "core people" will wither without direct, face-to-face communication that allows all to be fully present and available to each other. It's also important that we resolve conflicts and nurture these relationships.

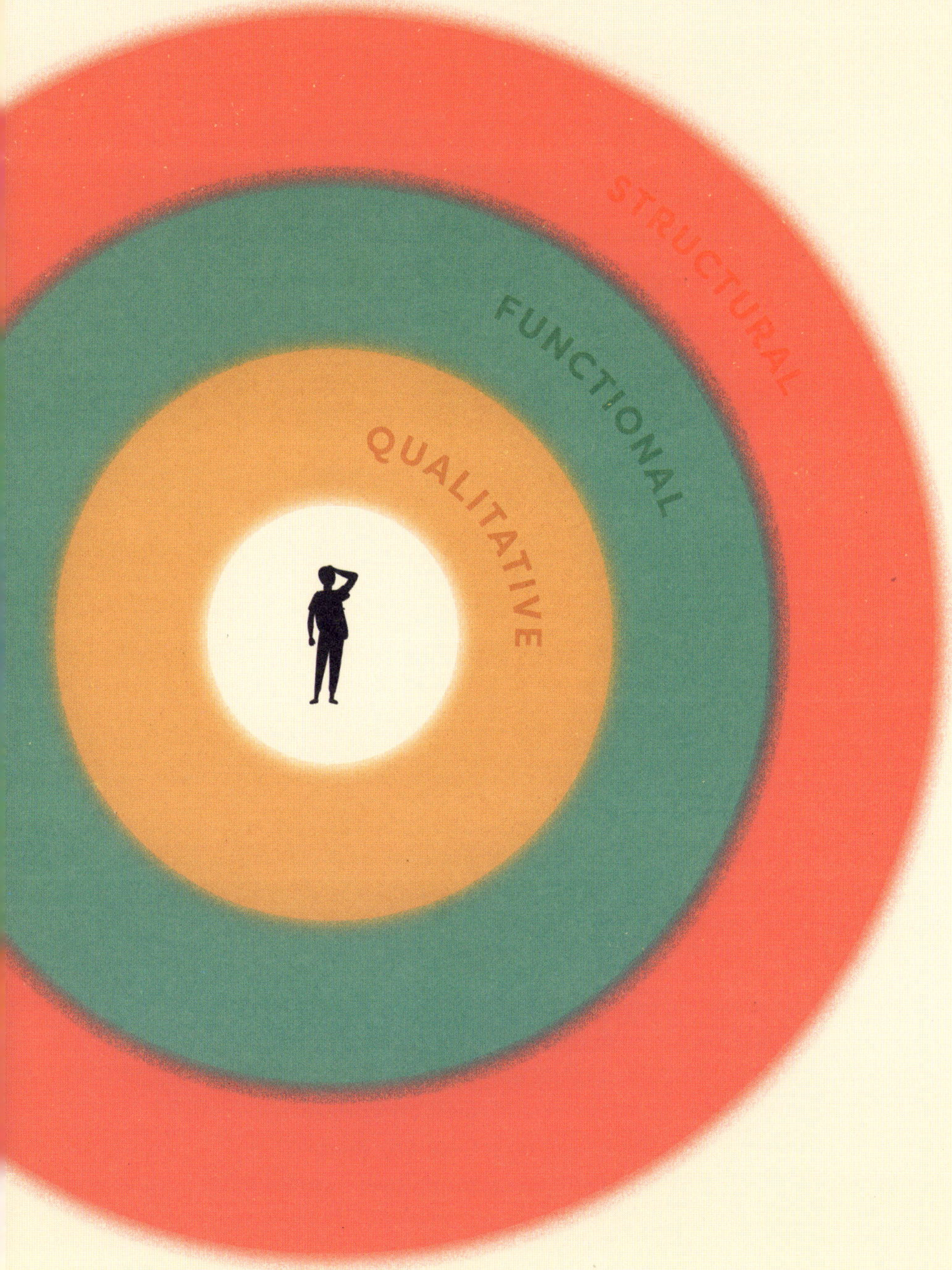
STRUCTURAL
FUNCTIONAL
QUALITATIVE

"A friend is one that knows you as you are, understands where you have been, accepts what you have become, and still, gently allows you to grow."

WILLIAM SHAKESPEARE

A LACK OF SOCIAL CONNECTION VERSUS LONELINESS

A lack of social connection is *objectively* having few or insufficient social relationships, social roles, and group memberships and thus experiencing infrequent social interaction. Loneliness is a distressing, *subjective*, internal state that results from perceived isolation or unmet needs between an individual's preferred and actual experience.

Who is in your inner circle? How are these relationships faring these days? Are you giving them your full attention and enough face-to-face time? In what ways do you need to strengthen these relationships?

THE THREE KINDS OF LONELINESS

Loneliness occurs when you lack sufficient social connections and you are, or feel, isolated physically or emotionally. Loneliness can also be classified into three main categories:

1. **Situational loneliness** occurs when life changes, such as moving away from friends and family or starting a new school or job, leaving you feeling isolated.

2. **Developmental loneliness** happens when you feel like you're falling behind in life compared to your peers, leading to feelings of isolation or low self-esteem.

3. **Internal loneliness** is when you feel alone in any and every situation, even when surrounded by people.

Identifying your type of loneliness can help you better understand and address the root cause. While situational loneliness may improve with time, developmental and internal loneliness often require more support and intervention. It's important to remember that loneliness is a universal feeling, and seeking help is a sign of strength, not weakness.

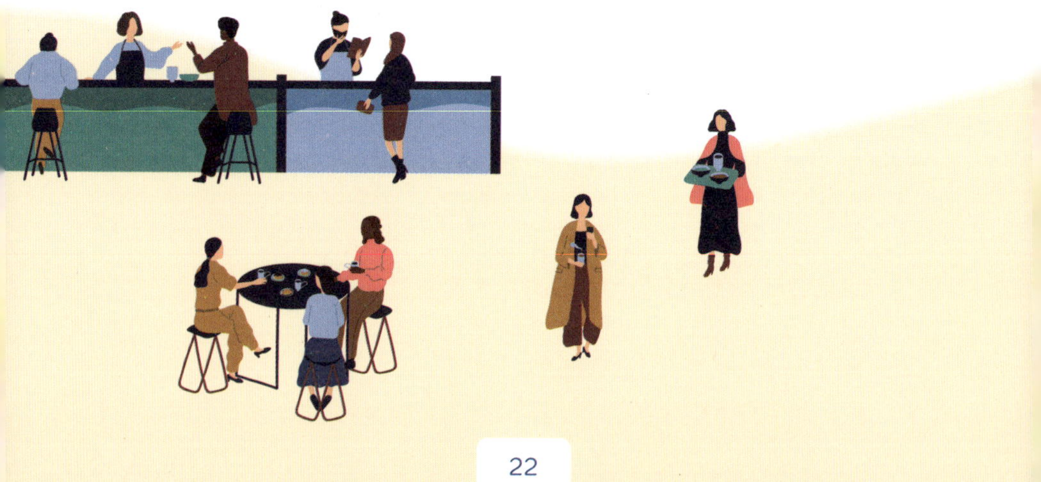

Situational loneliness is usually temporary and more easily fixed. One only needs to reach out to your new community or workplace. Be purposefully friendly and then ask someone to join you for lunch or drinks after work. Join a book club, a health club, a pickleball club, or take an art class, a swimming class, or a woodworking class. Find a church or a volunteer organization where you'd feel welcome. The point is that the sooner you reach out to make new friends, the sooner your situational loneliness will resolve itself.

List three activities you could sign up for to meet potential friends.

List three hobbies or activities you enjoy and three people you could ask to join you the next time you do them.

CONNECT EVERY DAY

To combat situational loneliness, make time for daily connection. Regular human interaction is key to combating and avoiding loneliness. Spend at least fifteen minutes every day talking with or writing to someone. Small, regular moments of connection—like checking in on a neighbor or asking someone how they're doing—add up. You can also chat with your local barista or the cashier in your local grocery store. Better yet, offer an act of kindness to a stranger. Simply being friendly will help you feel less lonely.

Developmental loneliness will require more effort. You may need to boost your self-esteem or even seek therapy. When you feel distanced due to feeling "less than," you are allowing your mind to convince you that others are doing better than you are. One way to combat this is to take a more realistic assessment of who you are.

Create a list of your top ten best qualities and call it "My Top Ten Attributes." Be generous in your assessment.

My Top Ten Attributes Are:

1

2

3

4

5

6

7

8

9

10

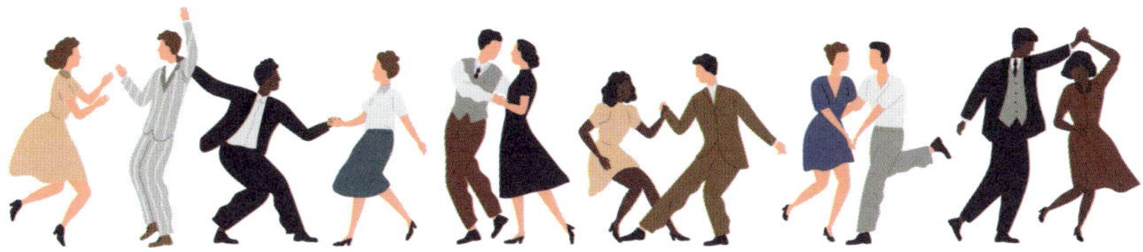

Compile a list of your top ten achievements in life. Call it "My Top Ten Achievements.

My Top Ten Achievements Are:

1

2

3

4

5

6

7

8

9

10

Also, create a list of attributes you ascribe to someone else that generates envy. It's highly possible that you already possess those same attributes and are simply projecting them onto someone else.

Attributes I most admire in someone else are:

Attributes I'd like to develop further include:

The point is that your mind can trick you into feelings that are not truly based on reality. We never truly know what others are going through, and it's highly likely that most feel as lonely and as inadequate as you do. Try observing more closely and offering others, and particularly yourself, more compassion.

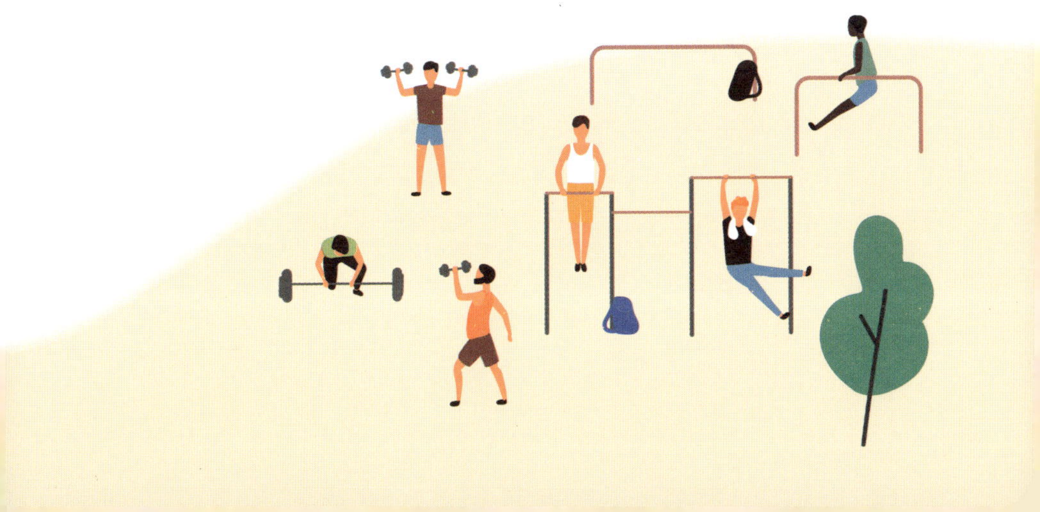

FORGIVE YOURSELF

We all tend to criticize and berate ourselves, which doesn't help us feel worthy of true connection. One way to feel more confident and worthy is to formally forgive yourself for whatever has made you feel inadequate, flawed, or "not enough." Choosing to forgive yourself removes the distance between your ideal self and your real self. In forgiving, you admit your failures, shortcomings, or faults and commit to your ideals.

Write a formal apology to yourself for whatever you perceive as grievous errors or failings. Write it as formally, detailed, and heartfelt as you would if writing a formal apology to a dear friend or family member. Be as clear and compassionate as possible. State what you did and why you're sorry. Also, include a promise that you will do better and commit to an improved relationship.

Once you've written your apology to yourself for perceived faults, shortcomings, or failures, stand in front of a mirror and read it aloud, looking up to meet your own eyes.

Example: *I apologize for not thinking more highly of myself and being more compassionate toward myself. I feel bad that I constantly underestimate and disappoint you, but I promise that I think very highly of you, that you are important to me, and that I will do better going forward. I know that you are likable and worthy of deep friendship. I value you and want to both win your trust and prove to you that you are very important to me. Please forgive me.*

Now write your apology:

INTERNAL LONELINESS

Where the cause of loneliness stems from internal factors, it's likely to impact your self-esteem negatively, creating a sense of inadequacy, self-blame, lowered self-worth, and even shame, all of which can make you withdraw even further from family and friends and thus become even lonelier. Loneliness can make you feel more apprehensive or fearful of social situations or pick up on what we view as social rejection cues too readily. If not addressed, internal loneliness may become embedded and lead us to view the cause of our loneliness as part of who we are.

While loneliness is not a mental health problem in itself, having mental health difficulties may lead to loneliness, which may then cause depression. Internal loneliness often involves depression, which means social interactions might temporarily distract but won't alleviate loneliness. Even when spending time with your partner or best friend, you might continue feeling listless, empty, and unable to engage.

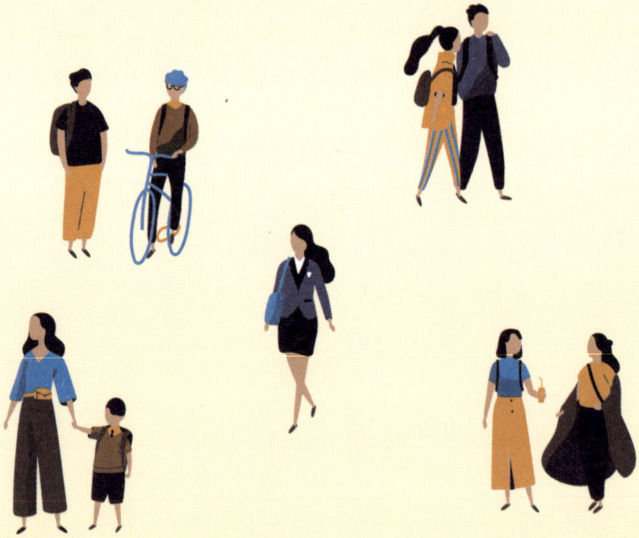

> “Where are the people?” resumed the little prince at last. “It’s a little lonely in the desert...”
>
> “It is lonely when you’re among people, too,” said the snake.”
>
> ANTOINE DE SAINT-EXUPÉRY,
> *THE LITTLE PRINCE*

CONNECT WITH YOURSELF

When you feel “less than” others and allow it to keep you from connecting with others, turn your attention inward. Instead of asking: Am I keeping up with whoever is in my social circles? Am I keeping up in a way that my mind says is comparable to others? Ask yourself: Am I being true to myself today? Have I been kind or a good friend to myself and others? Did I choose to act in ways consistent with what I value?” Then, give yourself credit for being true to yourself. Doing so will bolster a sense of self-efficacy, esteem, and comfort with who you are. Set aside at least five minutes a day (every day) to look inward and meditate, pray, practice yoga, or read a couple of pages of a spiritual text.

THE ROOT CAUSE OF INTERNAL LONELINESS

Internal loneliness can often be traced back to childhood experiences such as:

- Experiencing emotional or physical neglect
- Being made to feel like your feelings and needs didn't matter
- Being made to feel invisible because your parents were too busy to notice you
- Having to meet your emotional needs without support
- Not being seen, heard, and understood by your parents
- Not getting care, attention, and unconditional love.

Later in life, we find it hard to connect to others, to feel seen, and to feel heard, thus resulting in living with a constant feeling of loneliness and disconnection, whether you're surrounded by people or not.

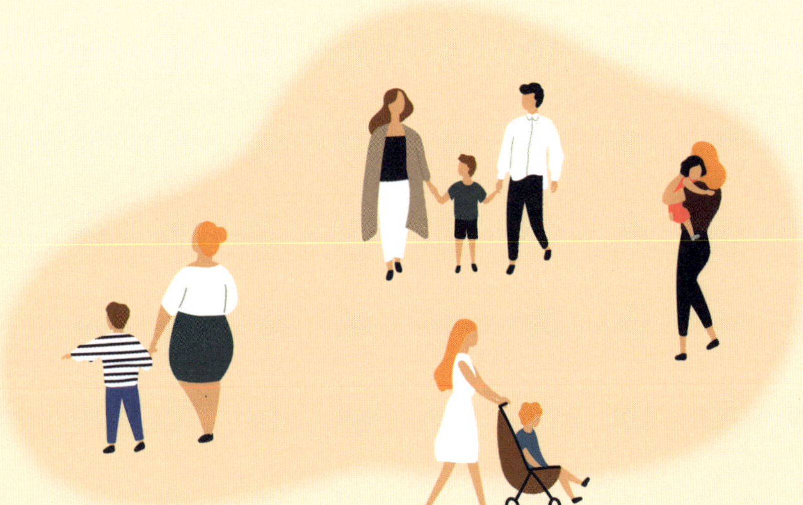

YES / NO	Did you experience emotional neglect as a child?
YES / NO	Did your parents punish or berate you for simply being you?
YES / NO	Did you often feel that your feelings and needs did not matter?
YES / NO	Were you often left on your own to cope with your emotions?
YES / NO	Did you feel misunderstood as a child?
YES / NO	Did you often feel rejected and hurt?
YES / NO	Did you often feel loved, nurtured, seen, and heard, then or now?

If the bulk of your answers are "yes," you may want to work with a therapist to address these types of deeply ingrained emotional wounds directly.

> "Severe separations in early life leave emotional scars on the brain because they assault the essential human connection: the [parent-child] bond which teaches us that we are lovable."
>
> JUDITH VIORST

COPING WITH INTERNAL LONELINESS

According to Kira Asatryan, relationship coach and author of *Stop Being Lonely*, even if you have close friends and family, internal loneliness occurs when you have very few people in your life you trust completely and with whom you can share your deepest concerns. Having close relationships buffers anxiety and depression because it lets you know that someone cares about you and limits the frustration and anger that comes when you feel as if no one understands you. These types of intimate relationships help you feel safe in the world and function at your peak capacity.

Asatryan recommends you foster intimacy by:

- Having deeper conversations with intimates
- Asking questions that foster closeness
- Finding unifying commonalities while also accepting differences
- Talking productively (positively) about your past and future
- Comfortably disclosing your inner world with others.

She says you achieve this by:

- Feeling and identifying your emotions
- Experiencing and offering empathy
- Bonding deeply with another without surrendering your identity
- Showing someone that you explicitly care about them
- Handling disagreements while still communicating caring
- Maintaining a reciprocal bond of caring over a long period.

Which of the previous suggestions can you implement in your life?

With whom can you start initiating changes in the way you interact?

Which suggestions will be more difficult?

Which people will present a greater challenge?

Throughout the rest of this book, we'll be discussing techniques that can help you address whichever type of loneliness you're experiencing. However, if you are also depressed or suffering from long-term loneliness, a counselor or therapist might be helpful in resolving past traumas and developing the kind of self-love and self-esteem needed to overcome them.

LONELINESS VERSUS SOLITUDE

It's important to note that being alone is not the same as being lonely. Loneliness occurs when someone desires social connection and intimacy but has difficulty finding it and feels isolated and disconnected as a result. It is often perceived as an involuntary separation, rejection, or abandonment by other people. Loneliness can be emotionally and even physically painful.

Solitude, however, is voluntary. People who enjoy spending time by themselves continue to maintain positive social relationships that they can easily access when they want a connection. People who enjoy and choose solitude balance interactions with others with periods alone. While research clearly shows that loneliness and isolation are bad for both mental and physical health, solitude has a number of important mental health benefits, including allowing people to better focus and recharge.

> "When I get lonely these days, I think: So, *be* lonely, Liz. Learn your way around loneliness. Make a map of it. Sit with it for once in your life. Welcome to the human experience. But never again use another person's body or emotions as a scratching post for your own unfulfilled yearnings."
>
> ELIZABETH GILBERT,
>
> *EAT, PRAY, LOVE*

Do you enjoy being alone? What makes that time productive or pleasurable?

How do your times of solitude compare to the times you feel lonely?

What kinds of activities can you pursue when alone that would make it more pleasurable?

ARE YOU AN INTROVERT OR AN EXTROVERT?

According to the founder of analytical psychology, Carl Jung, extroverts typically feel energized by being surrounded by people, enjoy interacting with the outside world, and prefer sharing their thoughts and feelings with others, while introverts typically feel recharged by being alone, feel most secure and confident in their own space, and like opportunities to contemplate quietly in a serene place. So, which are you? Answer "yes" or "no" to the following questions:

YES / NO	Do you enjoy spending time alone, focused on your thoughts?
YES / NO	Does being alone help you recharge?
YES / NO	Do you prefer activities or hobbies that take place in a small, quiet setting?
YES / NO	Does being at a crowded party make you uncomfortable?
YES / NO	Do you avoid meeting new people and feel drained after socializing?
YES / NO	Do you spend more time listening than talking?
YES / NO	Do you feel uncomfortable when the spotlight is on you?
YES / NO	Do you initiate conversations or wait for someone to talk to you?

YES / NO	Do you enjoy socializing with various kinds of people, most of whom you don't know?
YES / NO	Does being around other people, exploring new places, or experiencing lively environments make you feel energized?
YES / NO	Are you broad-minded, easy to approach, and comfortable in most social situations?
YES / NO	Do you find it easy to talk to almost anyone about almost anything?
YES / NO	Are you always game for a social outing?
YES / NO	Do you often initiate conversations with others?
YES / NO	Do you prefer to talk about yourself rather than listen to someone else ramble on?
YES / NO	Do you enjoy being the center of attention?

If you answered "yes" to questions 1–8, you are more introverted; and if you answered "yes" to questions 8–16, you are more extroverted, but being extroverted does not mean that you aren't lonely.

EVEN EXTROVERTS GET LONELY

Extroverts are often surrounded by others and may have many friends, but they may not form deep attachments. Also, because they love being around other people, tend to keep the spotlight on themselves, and derive both affirmation and energy from socializing, they may find being alone stressful. They may feel lonelier than introverts when alone. Contrary to what many may assume, because they are comfortable being alone with only their own thoughts, an introvert may not ever feel lonely.

INTROVERTS ARE SOCIAL BEINGS

Perhaps surprisingly, introverts may ultimately be the more social beings, because:

- They prefer having a smaller, select group of friends with whom they can share and discuss what's important to them, as well as their vulnerabilities.
- They socialize with fewer people, but once acquainted, introverts often form longer-lasting, more intimate relationships.
- They pay attention when others talk, avoid conflict, and think about their words and actions, which shows consideration for others.
- They take time to build friendships, invest more energy in forming attachments, and, once they establish mutual trust, offer a true, reciprocal friendship.

BEING AMBIVERT IS BEST

While there's nothing wrong with being an introvert or an extrovert, ideally, you want to be an ambivert, someone who has both introverted and extroverted attributes. Ambiverts:

- Feel energized when socializing, but also enjoy solitude.
- Are highly adaptable, flexible, and capable of striking a balanced social life.
- Both listen and speak well, making them compatible with introverts, extroverts, and other personality types.
- Are flexible in their thinking, tend to be good-natured, and are both empathetic and supportive.

As you proceed through this book, we'll discuss multiple ways to bolster social skills that will foster ambivert tendencies.

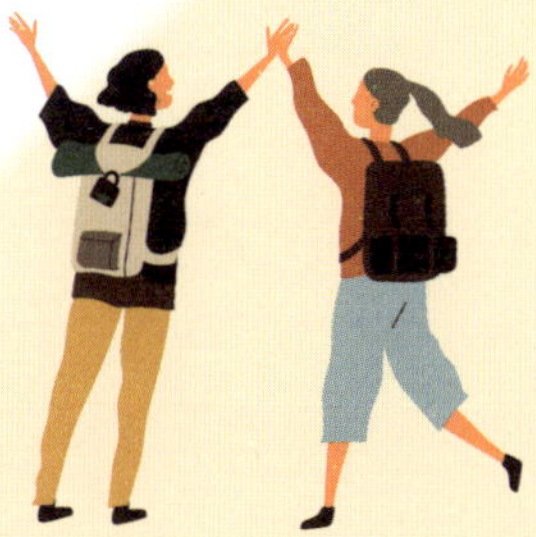

QUALITY TRUMPS QUANTITY

Research shows that you reap the psychological well-being and physical health benefits of social connection not from the number of friends you have but from the depth of your internal and subjective sense of connection toward others. It's the quality of your connections, not the number.

“But many of us seek community solely to escape the fear of being alone. Knowing how to be solitary is central to the art of loving. When we can be alone, we can be with others without using them as a means of escape.”

BELL HOOKS

ALL ABOUT LOVE: NEW VISIONS

CHAPTER 2

HOW LONELY ARE YOU?

As noted, even the loneliest people don't tend to view their condition as problematic. You could feel lonely often and still not recognize it as something you need to address. Let's take a quiz to see if you're lonelier than you think.

TAKE THE LONELINESS QUIZ

Answer the following "yes" or "no" questions. Do not include your spouse or significant other as a friend.

YES / NO Do you talk to someone daily?

YES / NO Are you often by yourself and bored?

YES / NO Does being alone make you anxious?

YES / NO Do you often feel out of sorts?

YES / NO Do you have friends with similar interests?

YES / NO Do you regularly make time to enjoy activities with friends?

YES / NO Do you have three or more close personal friendships in which you are truly authentic?

YES / NO Do you have long conversations with friends on a regular basis?

YES / NO Do you talk with friends in-depth about your personal issues?

YES / NO Are you close to your siblings or other family members?

YES / NO Do you make time to see family often?

YES / NO Do you offer them your full attention when present?

YES / NO Do you have close friends at work?

YES / NO Do you invite coworkers to socialize outside of work?

YES / NO Do you trust anyone at work with your secrets?

YES / NO Do you make new friends easily?

YES / NO Do you tend to avoid parties and other social events?

YES / NO Are you able to be vulnerable in relationships?

YES / NO Are you experiencing conflict in important relationships?

YES / NO Do you feel like your friends appreciate you?

YES / NO Do you have someone you feel truly understands you?

YES / NO If you are in an emotional crisis, do you have friends you can call?

YES / NO Do you have a faith-based community?

YES / NO Do you spend too much time isolated or alone?

YES / NO Would you rather be alone than with others?

Which of the previous questions most identified your problem areas?

Which of those are you most concerned about?

When you're feeling lonely, how do you comfort yourself? Is it effective?

If you're not reaching out to others to form deeper connections, why not?

RATE YOUR LEVEL OF LONELINESS

Now, in reviewing your answers, rate how lonely you are on a scale of one to four, with four being "I am problematically lonely," three being "I *definitely* need more people I love and trust in my life," two being "I need to expand my social circle and deepen my relationships"; and one being "I am occasionally lonely and need to make myself more vulnerable."

There is no perfect rating because we are all lonely sometimes, and it's highly likely that you're lonelier than you've even realized.

If you want to explore the depth of your loneliness more, you can find the Berkman-Syme Social Network Index: NIMH Data Archive – Data Dictionary: Data Structure (nih.gov) Or the UCLA Loneliness Scale: UCLA Loneliness Scale (Version 3) | SPARQtools.

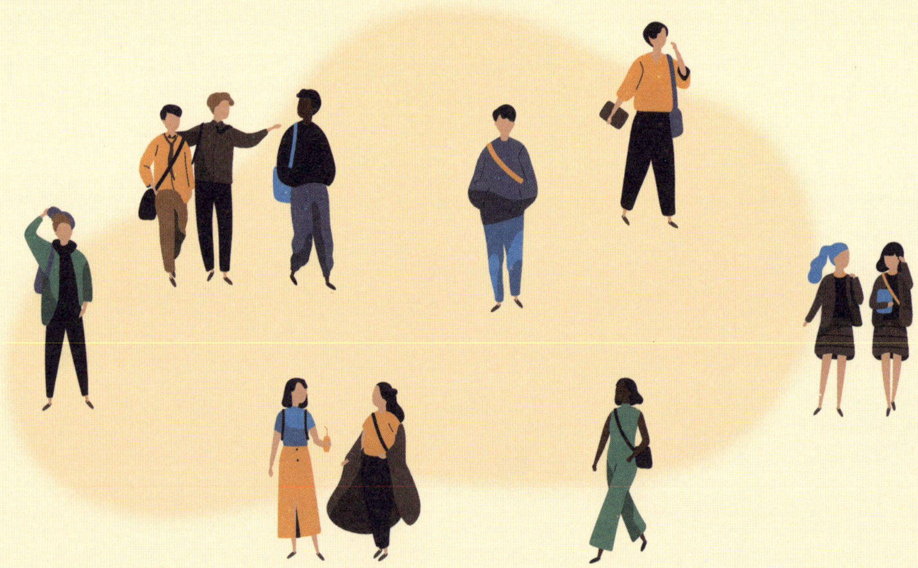

"The lonelier you are, the more you pull away until humans seem an alien race, with customs and a language you can't begin to understand."

ALICE HOFFMAN,

PRACTICAL MAGIC

SYMPTOMS ARE BELL WEATHERS

According to David Cates, PhD, director of behavioral health at Nebraska Medicine in Omaha, “Loneliness is like (physical) pain. It can be hard to measure, but you know when you feel it.” Recognizing physical symptoms caused by loneliness reminds you that you definitely need more quality time and genuine intimacy with friends and family.

Physical symptoms of loneliness might include:

- Bodily pain without an identifiable cause
- Headaches, migraines, stomach aches, or muscle tension
- Difficulty falling or staying sleeping
- Feeling fatigued
- Lack of appetite
- Feeling stressed out, sad, or depressed
- Difficulty focusing or poor decision-making
- Feeling foggy or experiencing memory problems
- Abusing food, alcohol, or drugs.

Are you experiencing any of these symptoms? Which ones? How long has this been happening?

Psychological signs of loneliness might include:

- Feeling hopeless, worthless, or increased feelings of depression
- Increased feelings of anxiety
- Excess shopping or increased attachment to material things
- Drinking more or using drugs
- Repeatedly binge-watching television
- Excessive reliance on social media.

YES, LONELINESS HURTS!

According to Elizabeth Scott, PhD on *verywellmind.com*, research shows that the areas of the brain that deal with social exclusion are the same areas that process physical pain, adding a scientific explanation to the often-romanticized experience of a "broken heart." If you're feeling emotional pain, take it seriously and proactively address the reasons.

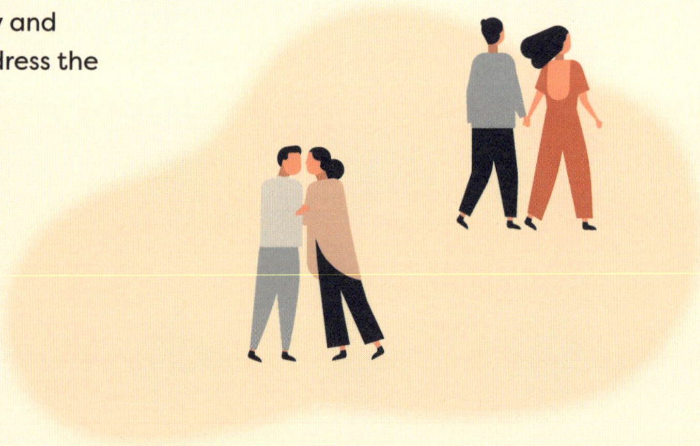

Are you experiencing any of the previous symptoms? How long has it been happening? Is this something you can address, or do you need to talk with your doctor?

"Solitude is the profoundest fact of the human condition. Man is the only being who knows he is alone."

OCTAVIO PAZ,

THE LABYRINTH OF SOLITUDE

IS IT YOUR ATTACHMENT STYLE?

Development psychologist Mary Ainsworth developed a theory that the attachments infants form with their primary caregiver affect their social, emotional, and cognitive development. When an infant's primary caregiver is available, sensitive, and responsive to the child's physical and emotional needs, the consistency of care helps the child feel safe in the world, which supports and encourages healthy development. Such children develop a secure attachment style. If the primary caretaker is not available, sensitive, and responsive, the child may form an insecure attachment rooted in difficult childhood bonding experiences. Your attachment style can then affect how you form attachments with others. Three types of insecure attachments result:

1. **An anxious-ambivalent attachment** style occurs when the primary caregiver is inconsistent in offering love and affection based on factors the child can neither predict nor understand. The parent typically leaves or withdraws love and affection without a reasonable explanation, which causes the infant to feel insecure. Future relationships are likely to be fraught with anxiety, resulting in clinging or controlling behavior.

2. **An anxious-avoidant attachment** occurs when a primary caregiver responds slowly or even neglects the infant's needs to such a degree that the infant learns to ignore his needs and self-soothe at an early age. These children may appear self-confident and self-sufficient later in life, but they tend to dismiss their emotional needs and tamp down their anxiety by avoiding relationships.

3. **A fearful-avoidant attachment** develops when a parent fails to respond appropriately or consistently to their child's feelings of fear or distress, often to the point of neglect or abuse. The parent may often respond in frustration or anger, which causes the child to grow up fearful and afraid to reveal his true emotions.

How do you think your relationships have been affected by your attachment style?

Early experiences with caregivers create an internal working model of social relationships, a system of thoughts, memories, beliefs, expectations, emotions, and behaviors about the self and others. It could be that your attachment style is hampering your ability to connect with others and form intimate relationships. To determine whether you're dealing with an insecure attachment disorder, answer "yes" or "no" to the questions below:

YES / NO Was your primary caregiver regularly available and responsive to your needs?

YES / NO Did either of your parents withhold love or withdraw without explanation?

YES / NO Did you often feel lonely as a child?

YES / NO Did you temper your behavior to avoid feeling unloved?

YES / NO Do you choose people you can trust as friends?

YES / NO Do you feel confident in your adult relationships?

YES / NO Do you form equal, reciprocal relationships, or are you always the giver?

If most of your answers are "yes," you may have an anxious-ambivalent attachment style.

YES / NO	Were you left on your own a lot as a small child?
YES / NO	Did you have a trustworthy caretaker who emanated love and concern?
YES / NO	Could you rely on either or both of your parents to take care of your basic needs?
YES / NO	Were you an anxious child? Clingy? Easily upset? Sad?
YES / NO	Did you feel safe and loved as a child?
YES / NO	Do you isolate yourself in an effort to manage anxiety?
YES / NO	Do you tend to push people away or sabotage relationships?

If most of your answers are "yes," you may have an anxious-avoidant attachment style.

YES / NO	Were either of your primary caregivers abusive?
YES / NO	Did you often feel unsafe in your home environment?
YES / NO	Were you often neglected? Hungry? Lonely? Fearful?
YES / NO	Did you have to protect yourself from someone's out-of-control behavior?
YES / NO	Does a fear of intimacy keep you from forming relationships?
YES / NO	Do you feel that you have to hide parts of yourself?
YES / NO	Are you too passive in relationships?

If most of your answers are "yes," you may have a fearful-avoidant attachment style.

THE CUMULATIVE EFFECT

Depending upon how you respond to feeling alone and the actions you take to address it, loneliness often has a cumulative effect on how you feel and behave, either spiraling down toward deeper loneliness or spiraling up toward stronger connections. Here's how both spirals work:

DOWNWARD SPIRAL

Personal circumstances, a precipitating event, or both leave you feeling alone.

Low self-esteem; negative thoughts and feelings about yourself.

Distancing yourself from others.

Increased negativity, a feeling of despair.

Further withdrawal from relationships; more time spent alone.

Severe loneliness.

UPWARD SPIRAL

Increased engagement with others.

Changing how you relate to others.

Experiencing a shift in thoughts and feelings, accompanied by faith in positive change.

Learning how to challenge automatic thoughts and feelings by observing, addressing, and reframing them.

Recognizing that these unchallenged negative thoughts and feelings created ingrained patterns of behavior.

Realizing that your thoughts and feelings related to loneliness have influenced how you behave around others.

"Loneliness watches and sighs, then climbs into my bed and pulls the covers over himself, fully dressed, shoes and all. He's going to make me sleep with him again tonight, I just know it."

ELIZABETH GILBERT,

EAT, PRAY, LOVE

CHAPTER 3

TAME YOUR DIGITAL OBSESSION

Digital technologies are pervasive in our lives. Nearly all American teens and adults under sixty-five (96–99 percent) and 75 percent of adults sixty-five and over use the internet and spend an average of six hours per day on digital media. One in three US adults eighteen and over report that they are online "almost constantly," and the percentage of teens ages thirteen to seventeen years who say they are online "almost constantly" has doubled since 2015. Regarding social media specifically, the percentage of US adults eighteen and over who reported using social media increased from 5 percent in 2005 to roughly 80 percent in 2019. Among teens ages thirteen to seventeen years, 95 percent report using social media as of 2022, with more than half reporting it would be hard to give up social media.

Telephones and social media aren't the worst—or the only—deterrent to true social connection, but if you want to expand your social circle and deepen all your personal relationships, taming your digital obsession is a great place to start, and dependent on your usage, an essential place to start.

> "Texts, emails, Facebook pokes, and Twitter faves do not a social life make. People are, it would seem, lonelier than ever, and also less used to being alone."
>
> LENA DUNHAM

ARE YOU SOCIAL-MEDIA OBSESSED?

Spending a lot of time scrolling on social media accelerated one of the newest neuroses: the FOMO phenomenon (fear that you are missing out on something fundamentally important). Seeing highlights of what looks like the fabulous lives other people are living not only leads you to feel as if you're missing out or falling short, but it also creates a sense of social competition, which leads to a false sense of what "normal" is. Research shows that a fear of missing out can stem from unhappiness and dissatisfaction with life. These feelings can propel us into greater social media usage, which, in turn, can make us feel worse about ourselves and our lives, not better. Excessive social media consumption becomes a vicious cycle that needs to be broken.

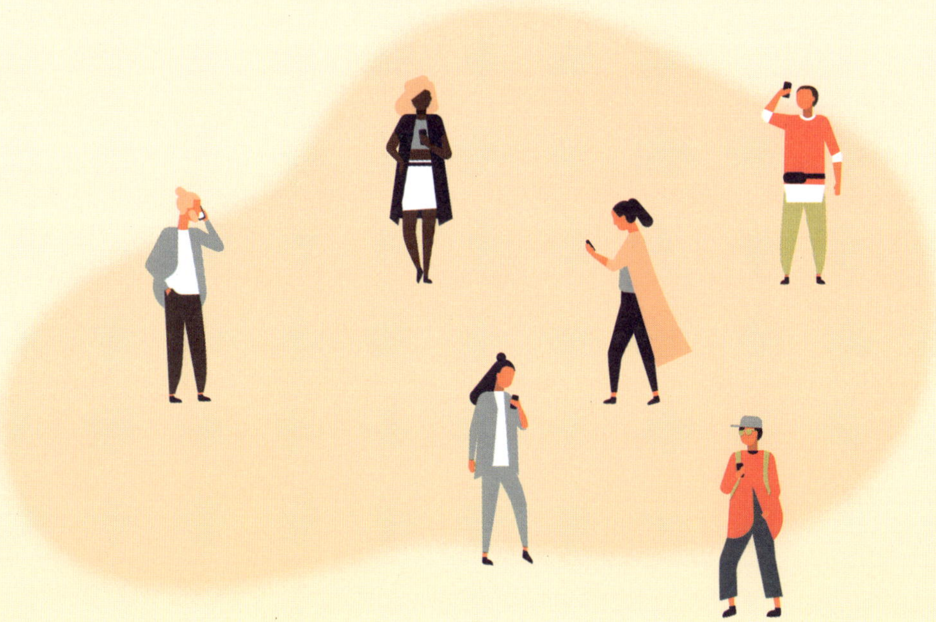

How much time do you spend each day scrolling on social media?

Are you often envious of what appears to be more exciting lives?

Does seeing other people's posts make you feel "less than" or as if you're missing out?

Do your friends and family complain that you pay more attention to your phone than them?

Do you turn off (or completely ignore) your phone when socializing?

"When was the last time you were dazzled? When was the last time you lay down on a block of granite and fell asleep beneath the sky? Our few remaining pockets of unconnected, unwired time are dwindling fast."

ANTHONY DOERR

HAS IT BECOME A BEHAVIORAL ADDICTION?

Many experts believe that tech and device overuse may become a behavioral addiction that can lead to physical, psychological, and social problems. In a poll conducted by Common Sense Media, 50 percent of teens reported feeling addicted to their mobile devices, and 78 percent of teen respondents checked their digital devices hourly. Researchers in Sweden found that heavy technology use among young adults was linked to sleeping problems, depressive symptoms, and increased stress levels.

You may have a **behavioral addiction** to your phone if you:

- Spend the majority of your time engaged in, thinking about, or arranging to engage in the behavior
- Depend on the behavior to cope with emotions or "feel normal"
- Neglect work, school, or family to engage in the behavior more often
- Minimize or hide the extent of your problem
- Continue despite physical or mental harm
- Experience symptoms of withdrawal (depression or irritability) when trying to stop.

If you are struggling with a behavioral addiction that is adversely affecting your health or quality of life, talk with your health provider about treatment options. The questions on the next page may indicate a problem.

YES / NO Have you turned off notifications on social media sites?

YES / NO Are you comfortable doing so now?

YES / NO Do you limit your time on social media?

YES / NO Could you easily decrease current usage by half?

YES / NO Shortly thereafter, can you adhere to a schedule that involves checking social media once or twice a day for no more than fifteen minutes?

YES / NO Have you ever gone more than five hours without checking your phone?

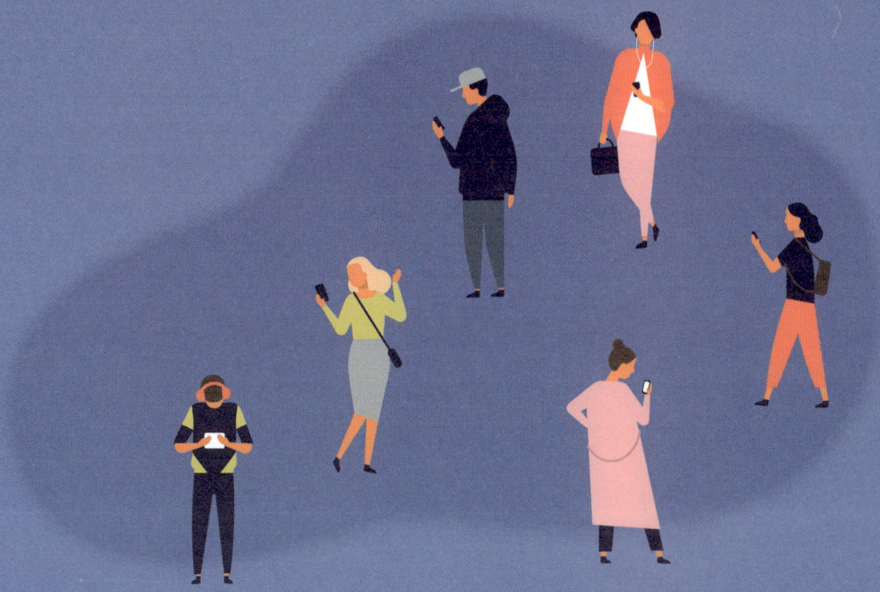

How did you feel answering the questions on the previous page?

How do you feel after spending long periods of time on your phone?

“People are so lonely, they spend their birthdays on the internet thanking people for wishing them a happy birthday, people who only know it’s their birthday because Facebook told them.”

CAROLINE KEPNES,

HIDDEN BODIES

TRY DIGITAL DETOX

Kendra Cherry, author of Everything Psychology, identified these signs that you are likely addicted to your phone and definitely need digital detox:

- You feel anxious or stressed out if you can't find your phone
- You feel compelled to check your phone every few minutes
- You feel depressed, anxious, or angry after spending time on social media
- You are preoccupied with the like, comments, or reshare counts on your social posts
- You're afraid that you'll miss something if you don't keep checking your device
- You often find yourself staying up late or getting up early to play on your phone
- You have trouble concentrating on one thing without having to check your phone.

You can initiate digital detox by pushing all unnecessary notifications and choosing one or two specific times when you'll spend only twenty to thirty minutes reading nonessential texts, news, or social posts. If you need your devices for your job, pick a time when you can turn off your devices, and then focus on spending an evening completely free of things like social media, texting, online videos, and other electronic distractions.

- To further detox, strictly avoid cellphone usage:
- When you first wake up or before breakfast
- When you eat meals, particularly with other people
- When you want to focus on a project or hobby
- When you visit with friends or family in person
- Two hours before you go to sleep each night.

Once you've seen the benefits of limiting phone usage, consider leaving your phone at home whenever possible.

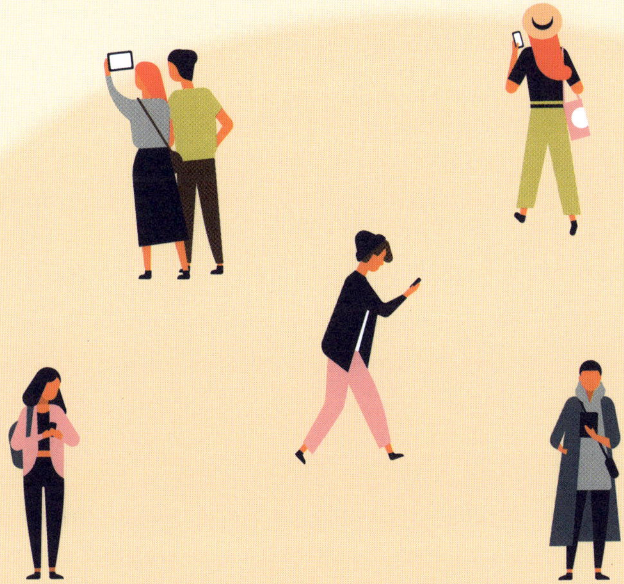

List three ways you can immediately detox from excessive phone usage or social media engagement.

1

2

3

THIRTY MINUTES TOPS!

In a 2018 study reported in the *Journal of Social and Clinical Psychology*, researchers from the University of Pennsylvania recently linked the use of social media sites such as Facebook, Snapchat, and Instagram to decreased well-being. The results revealed that limiting social media exposure to thirty minutes a day decreased symptoms of depression and loneliness.

"It has been said that people of the modern world suffer a great sadness, a 'species loneliness'—estrangement from the rest of Creation. We have built this isolation with our fear, with our arrogance, and with our homes brightly lit against the night."

ROBIN WALL KIMMERER,

BRAIDING SWEETGRASS

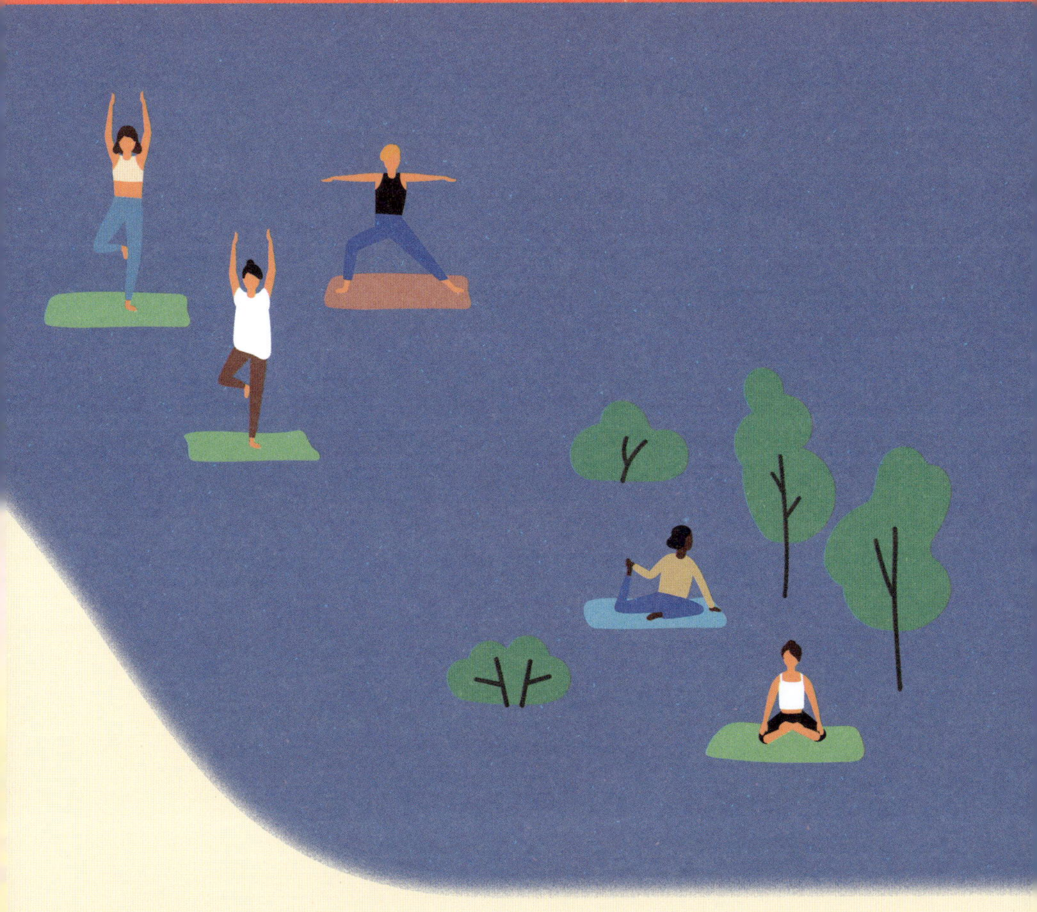

“A great fire burns within me, but no one stops to warm themselves at it, and passers-by only see a wisp of smoke”

VINCENT VAN GOGH

CHAPTER 4

IMPROVE YOUR SELF-ESTEEM

Self-esteem plays a huge role in how you view yourself and how you live your life. Some of the consequences of low self-esteem are an increased likelihood of being or feeling isolated and removed, a limited social life, and difficulty connecting on deep levels. Healthy self-esteem fosters your ability to form social connections and intimate relationships.

SIGNS THAT YOU HAVE HEALTHY SELF-ESTEEM ARE:

- You don't dwell on past negative experiences
- You believe you are equal to others, no better and no worse
- You comfortably express your needs
- You feel confident
- You maintain a positive outlook on life
- You say "no" when you want to
- You see your overall strengths and weaknesses and accept them.

Healthy self-esteem helps you navigate life knowing that you are capable of accomplishing what you set your mind to. It also helps you set appropriate relationship boundaries and maintain a healthy relationship with yourself and others.

SIGNS THAT YOU HAVE LOW SELF-ESTEEM ARE:

- You view others as better than you
- You have difficulty expressing your needs
- You focus on your weaknesses
- You are plagued by fear, self-doubt, and worry
- You have a negative outlook on life and feel a lack of control
- You harbor an intense fear of failure
- You struggle to accept positive feedback
- You have trouble saying "no" and setting boundaries
- You put other people's needs before your own
- You lack confidence.

With low self-esteem, you may find it difficult to pursue your goals and maintain healthy relationships, which can negatively impact your quality of life and increase the likelihood of experiencing anxiety and episodic or chronic depression.

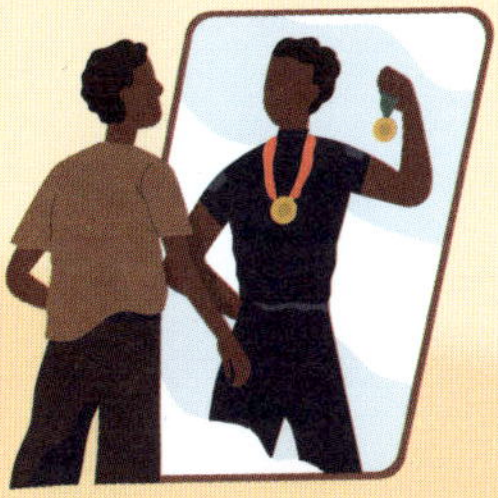

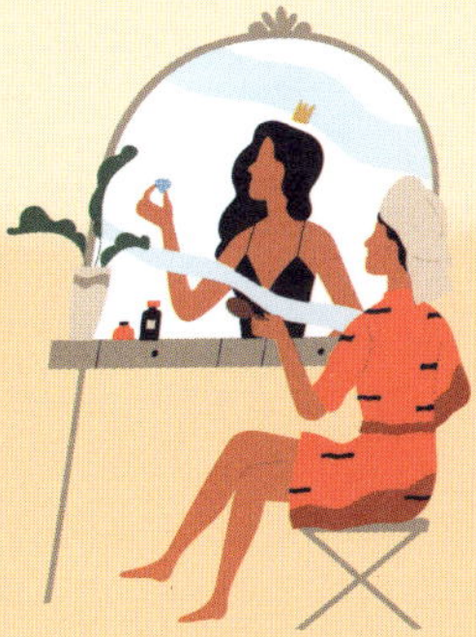

In reviewing the two lists, where would you rank yourself on these qualities? Do you have more checkmarks on the high or low list? Presuming everyone experiences low self-esteem occasionally, make a list of the issues you need to address to bolster your self-esteem.

“True belonging only happens when we present our authentic, imperfect selves to the world; our sense of belonging can never be greater than our level of self-acceptance. True belonging doesn’t require you to *change* who you are. It requires you to *be* who you are.”

BRENÉ BROWN

YOU CAN HAVE TOO MUCH SELF-ESTEEM

Overly high self-esteem is often mislabeled as narcissism. However, individuals with narcissistic traits may only *appear* to have high self-esteem. Their self-esteem may appear high or low but, in reality, is unstable, constantly shifting depending on the given situation. You can have excessive self-esteem and not be a narcissist.

SIGNS YOU HAVE TOO MUCH SELF-ESTEEM ARE:

- You may be preoccupied with being perfect
- You may focus on always being right
- You may believe you cannot fail
- You may believe you are more skilled or better than others
- You may express grandiose ideas
- You may grossly overestimate your skills and abilities

When self-esteem is too high, it can result in relationship problems, difficulty with social situations, and an inability to accept criticism.

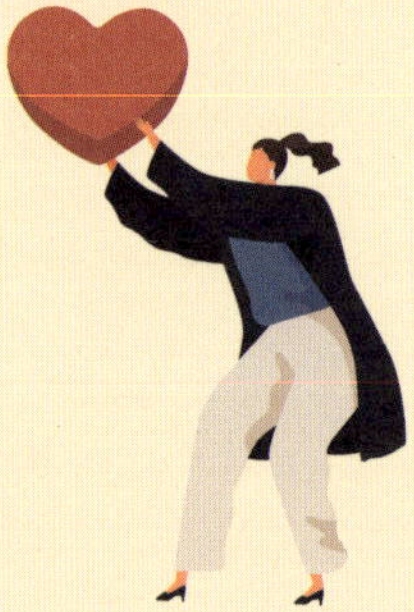

YES / NO — Do you have far better knowledge or savvy than most of your contemporaries?

YES / NO — Do you have a genuine interest in what other people have to say?

YES / NO — Have you ever been accused of being condescending or impatient?

YES / NO — Do you give others their due and see them as equally intelligent, attractive, and charismatic?

YES / NO — Do you secretly feel superior to most of the people you meet?

YES / NO — Do you feel smarter than most of your workmates?

YES / NO — Is it possible your self-esteem is so high that others keep you at arm's distance because you come across as smug or all-knowing?

If any of your answers are "yes," you may want to tamper your image of yourself with a hearty dose of reality, tone down self-love, and develop more compassion and generosity toward others.

BOOST YOUR SELF-ESTEEM

If your self-esteem needs a boost before you address your loneliness, here are ways you can feel better about yourself:

- **Identify all the qualities** you possess that make you worthy and likable and someone others would benefit from knowing.
- **Identify any negative or distorted thoughts** you hold that impact your self-worth. Assess how valid these may or may not be. Typically, self-distortion is holding you back.
- **Disrupt negative thinking patterns** by countering those thoughts with more realistic or positive ones. Anytime you catch yourself thinking negative thoughts, flip the switch to a positive interpretation.
- **Use positive self-talk.** Create and use positive affirmations that support you. Be as emotionally supportive to yourself as you would to someone you love.
- **Practice self-compassion.** Practice forgiving yourself for past mistakes and moving forward by accepting all parts of yourself. We are all human and worthy of understanding, forgiveness, and compassion.

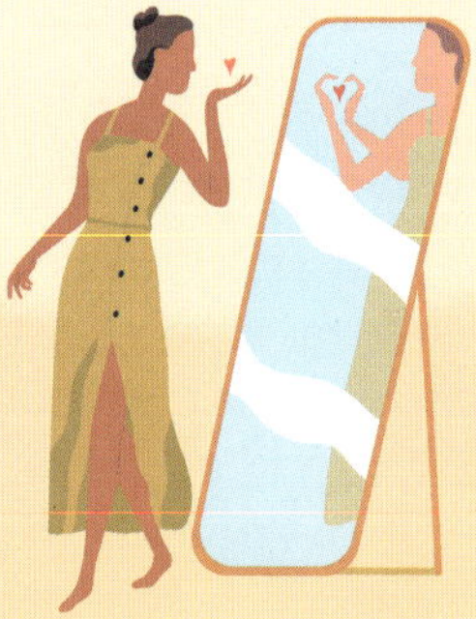

List the qualities that make you worthy and likable and someone others would benefit from knowing.

List any distorted or negative thoughts about yourself that you think or say. And then counter each of these thoughts with something that is both positive and far more likely to be true.

Write three to five positive affirmations that would help you like yourself more.

Write down anything you think needs to be forgiven, then write a sentence for each that expresses your forgiveness.

"As your mind grows quieter and more spacious, you can begin to see self-defeating thought patterns for what they are and open up to other, more positive options."

SHARON SALZBERG

TAKE SELF-APPRECIATION BREAKS

Take two minutes every day to seriously ponder *three things* that you can officially appreciate about yourself. Write them down in clear, positively stated sentences, then allow yourself to fully absorb these true statements, thereby giving yourself credit for these noteworthy traits.

CHALLENGE NEGATIVE THOUGHTS

How you talk to yourself and how you view a stressful situation can change when your self-esteem feels threatened. Your thoughts and beliefs might be positive, negative, or neutral. They might be rational, based on reason or facts, or they may be irrational, based on false ideas. Often, they are self-critical and self-defeating.

When caught up in stressful situations, notice what you say (or think) about yourself and how you view the situation, then ask yourself if your thoughts and observations are fair and true. Would you say them to a friend? If you wouldn't say them to someone else, *don't* say them to yourself.

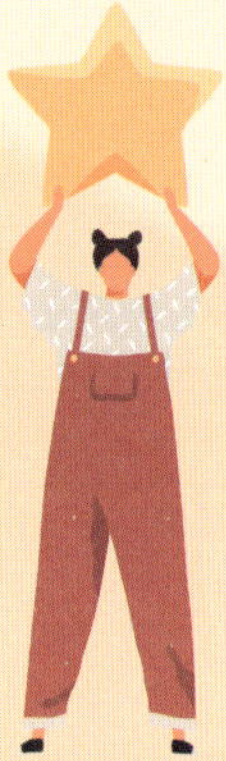

To help you begin developing an honest and realistic conception of yourself, list ten strengths you need to appreciate more.

1

2

3

4

5

6

7

8

9

10

List ten weaknesses you would like to change.
Be as objective as possible.

1

2

3

4

5

6

7

8

9

10

"The most oppressive feature of loneliness is the way it limits imagination, whispering to us that life will never be better, that we are not allowed to envision possibilities. Loneliness chips away at the space we occupy."

MAYA SHANBHAG LANG

DISRUPT NEGATIVE THOUGHT PATTERNS

Sometimes, your mind plays tricks on you, effectively putting a spin on events you see and attaching a subjective, rather than objective, interpretation to what you experience. These cognitive distortions are simply patterns of thinking or believing you may have adopted without scrutiny. You can counteract these thoughts and patterns by making them conscious and deliberately changing the way you process thoughts, observations, and experiences.

You likely don't realize how often you say negative things in your head or how much it affects how you interact with others. The first step to disrupt negative thought patterns is to notice how often they happen. Once you've increased awareness of your negative thought patterns, try the following techniques to disrupt them:

1. **Try thought-stopping.** Anytime you notice a negative thought or response, instruct yourself to "stop." If feasible, say it aloud, but if not, silently think it. If you're diligent, over time, you can break an unconscious pattern.

2. **Use the rubber band snap.** If necessary, try wearing a rubber band around your wrist, and each time you engage in negative self-talk, pull the band away from your skin and let it snap back. The sting will both bring attention to the pattern and disrupt it.

3. **Restate what you say and change how you think.** As soon as you notice a negative thought, immediately change it to a neutral or positive thought.

Are you often plagued with negative thoughts about yourself or about certain situations? What do you often think or say about yourself that is harsh, cruel, or simply unfair?

Take the most potent negative thoughts and reframe them in a compassionate manner. What do you know about yourself that counteracts such unfair negativity?

"It's how I fill the time when nothing's happening. Thinking too much, flirting with melancholy."

TIM WINTON,

BREATH

EMBRACE POSITIVE SELF-TALK

When faced with a situation that generates fear, such as meeting new people, try repeating positive affirmations that acknowledge your negative thoughts or emotions, then let them go.

EXAMPLES MIGHT INCLUDE:

Anxiety isn't dangerous. Despite feeling uncomfortable, I'm fully capable of dealing with whatever happens. I choose to overrule my anxiety and push myself to make new friends.

What I've been picturing isn't an objective assessment. I've been focused on potential negative aspects. I choose to focus on the positive possibilities of reaching out.

Yes, I'm feeling anxious, but so what? I'm familiar with anxiety, know it's based on distorted thoughts, and that it will pass. I'm choosing to be more social.

It's important that the statements you are making are realistic and true statements that are also positive. If they are not, your subconscious mind will know you're lying to yourself, which can actually trigger more anxiety.

Think back to the last time anxiety prevented you from doing something you wanted to do, particularly when it involved social connection. What negative thoughts were you having?

What did you postulate about yourself or the potential situation that caused anxiety? List the negative thoughts, and then reframe these thoughts in a far more balanced, fair way.

"You are the sky.
Everything else—
it's just the weather."

PEMA CHODRON

FOCUS ON HAPPY TIMES

Actively focusing on the positive and developing a sense of optimism can benefit your sense of well-being and serve as a coping mechanism. It can be as simple as identifying what brings pleasure in your current situation, as well as remembering the happiest times in your past. Take a moment to make a list of the happiest times in your life, particularly those in which you felt especially connected to others. When you feel lonely, spend a few minutes remembering one of those occasions, calling up as much detail as you can remember.

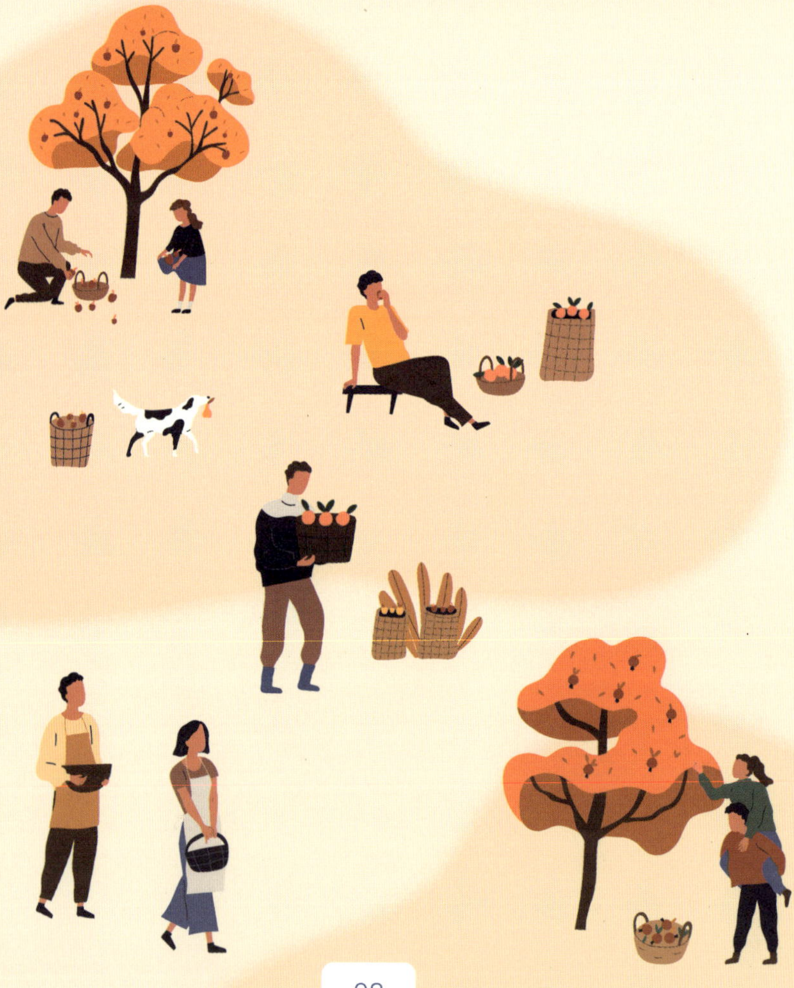

Create a list of happy times.

PRACTICE SELF-COMPASSION

Self-compassion is more than simply being kind to yourself. When practiced, it improves how you relate to yourself in a way that allows you to become more emotionally flexible, navigate challenging emotions, and enhance your connection to self and others. Dr. Kristin Neff, a psychologist and researcher in the area of self-compassion, suggests the following ways to practice self-compassion:

- **Imagine talking to a friend.** When going through a difficult time, take a moment to consider how you might respond to a close friend if they were going through a similar situation. Be as attentive, kind, and caring toward yourself as you would be to a dear friend.
- **Stop and observe.** Instead of reacting and trying to emotionally survive a distressing situation, slow down long enough to objectively observe your experience. Looking at the bigger picture will help keep things in perspective and help you see important information that may have been missed otherwise.
- **Change your self-talk.** Notice how you talk to yourself when you're experiencing negative emotions. Reframe your critical self-appraisals to more positive, nurturing ones. Picture yourself serving as a mentor or advocate to yourself, as opposed to a critic or judge.
- **Get clear on what you want.** When you reframe critical thoughts into more nurturing self-talk, it reveals clues as to what you need and want. Clarifying these needs will help you focus on where you want to go and what you are working toward, helping to increase motivation and happiness.
- **Care for yourself.** Recognize that your needs deserve to be met and that you are worthy of practicing self-care. The more you practice, the more you lessen the desire to engage in unhealthy coping behaviors when faced with challenges and stress.

Think back to the last time you came down hard on yourself for not doing something well. Write a sentence that expresses more compassion than judgment, "speaking" to yourself as you would a dear friend.

Think back to the last time you lost control of your emotions. Did you jump to the wrong conclusions? Were you overreacting? In looking at the bigger picture, what was really happening? What was really true?

Think back to the last time you were angry with yourself. Did you judge yourself harshly? Did you truly deserve a lashing? How would you "speak" to yourself with more compassion now?

Think about a way that you repeatedly judge and berate yourself for something. How can you rephrase any negative thoughts about what you lacked into a clear statement of how that anger may reflect what you *truly* want?

Write down three ways you can do something just for yourself in the coming weeks. Make it things that will leave you feeling special, nurtured, and loved.

OWN IT, THEN WRITE IT OUT

Take time each day to write about the challenges you are experiencing. Notice any self-critical statements or when you begin to feel alone in your experiences. As you would with self-talk, intentionally reframe any critical statements with a softer, more understanding tone to see—and, more importantly, *feel*—how the way you think and talk about yourself affects your ability to feel worthy and likable.

"There is no surer way to locate your self if you have misplaced her for a moment than to ask your*self* what you want."

RUFI THORPE

CHAPTER 5

EXPAND YOUR COMFORT LEVEL

TRY NEW THINGS

If it feels overwhelming to reach out to strangers or even to make yourself more vulnerable to people you do know, here are ways you can ease your way into being more social:

- **Talk to people** you encounter in your everyday life. Chat with cashiers at the grocery store or your server at lunch, and rather than simply wave, engage in conversation with neighbors. Remind yourself that you're a social being.
- **Go to places** where lots of people will be milling around, such as coffee shops, libraries, or bookstores. It's far better than remaining at home alone, where no opportunities for face-to-face interactions exist. Even just being around others decreases loneliness.
- Repeatedly, **go somewhere you feel comfortable** and linger there. Eventually, you'll recognize those who also frequent it, and eventually, you, or they, may find a reason to talk. When it happens, stay engaged and enjoy all the good feelings that result.
- **Join online forums.** Pick a topic that fascinates you, and you may find it easier to join in the conversation. Keep doing this until you feel comfortable being seen and talking.
- **Sign up for online classes.** Pick something you want to explore among people who may feel like your tribe, and your enthusiasm will help you risk being seen and heard.

As your comfort levels increase, push yourself to keep trying new things.

List three places you could go just to be around people.

1

2

3

List three places where you could “hang out” for hours and perhaps talk to someone.

1

2

3

List three online forums you could join.

1

2

3

List three online classes you could pursue. Make them something you want to explore.

1

2

3

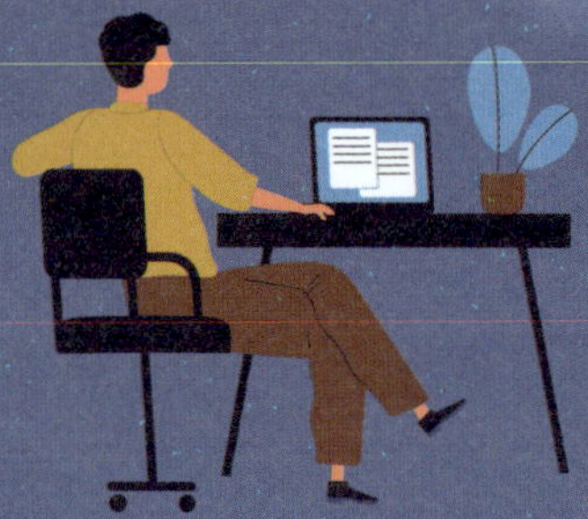

"A person is not supposed to go through life with absolutely nobody. It's not normal. The longer you go by yourself, the weirder you get, and the weirder you get, the longer you go by yourself. It's a loop, and you gotta do something to get out of it."

JIM SHEPARD

TRACK YOUR MOODS

Each day, go somewhere and make a concerted effort to expand your comfort level. Then, take notice of how any outreach makes you feel by creating the following journal entry.

Today I spent three hours at the library, where I smiled at everyone and initiated a conversation with two people for an extended length of time.

Before making a conscious effort to connect, I felt lonely, sad, sluggish, awkward, depressed, unworthy.

After connecting, however briefly, I felt joyful, centered, connected, friendly, uplifted, likable, approachable.

The more you notice how expanding your comfort level benefits your moods, the more you're likely to reach out to others.

Today I:

Before making a conscious effort to connect, I felt:

After connecting, however briefly, I felt:

BEFRIEND YOURSELF FIRST

Improving our relationships with ourselves, as well as others can help us feel less lonely. Here are a few ideas for befriending yourself:

- **Decide what self-care means to you.** Some people who live alone find it comforting to have some background noise. If that's you, it could be the television, the radio, or a podcast you enjoy. If you prefer quiet, turn it all off and relish the silence.
- **Do activities you enjoy by yourself.** Go for a walk to enjoy local landscaping, do your favorite arts or crafts, cook a meal from scratch, or start by simply moving your body, watching a film you love, decluttering your home, or going to a local museum.
- **Try different things to see what makes you feel good.** Experiment to find out what you can truly enjoy doing alone. Try something you've never done before.
- **Be patient with yourself.** It might feel weird at first, but stick with it, and soon you'll feel more comfortable just being *you*, by yourself, having fun.

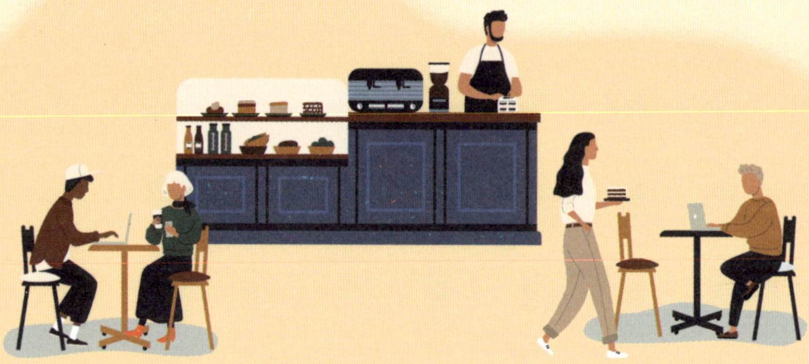

"Friendship is so weird. You just pick a human you've met, and you're like, 'Yep, I like this one,' and you just do stuff with them."

BILL MURRAY

IMPROVE YOUR SOCIAL SKILLS

Emotional intelligence is essential to fostering connection, and it's a skill you can develop. Here are six ways you can bolster your emotional intelligence, improve your social skills, and foster connection:

1. **Respond rather than react to conflict.** Rather than react to someone else's out-of-control emotions or behavior, take a moment to calm your own emotions. Once you feel calm, focus on finding a resolution, then keep your words and actions in alignment with your goal to defuse anger and foster understanding.

2. **Employ active listening skills.** Focus on what the other person is saying while also noticing nonverbal clues to what they might be feeling. Make sure you understand what is being said before responding and repeat what they said if you aren't sure. This prevents misunderstandings, allows the listener to respond properly, and shows respect for the other person.

3. **Maintain a positive attitude.** Be aware of and sensitive to other people's moods, but hold firm to your own. Don't allow someone else's negativity to invade your happy space. Do your best always to project a positive attitude. Do your best to uplift those around you.

4. **Practice self-awareness.** While remaining aware of your emotions, observe and intuit others' emotions and body language, then use that information to improve communication. Be aware of any nonverbal cues you may be sending, and make sure they reflect your true feelings.

5. **Empathize with others.** Even if you disagree with someone, do your best to feel what they feel and see it from their point of view. Empathy opens the door for mutual respect and understanding between people with differing opinions and situations.

6. **Be approachable and sociable.** Smile and radiate a positive presence. Maintain a welcoming attitude and people will be drawn to you.

Do you often feel socially awkward? Have others accused you of being socially awkward, insensitive, abrupt, dismissive, self-centered, or rude? What problem areas do you need to address?

Have people commented on your lack of social skills or accused you of falling short when it comes to being social? What do you specifically need to work on?

Is anxiety preventing you from connecting? What might be behind that anxiety? Are some situations more stressful than others? How can you make them more amenable?

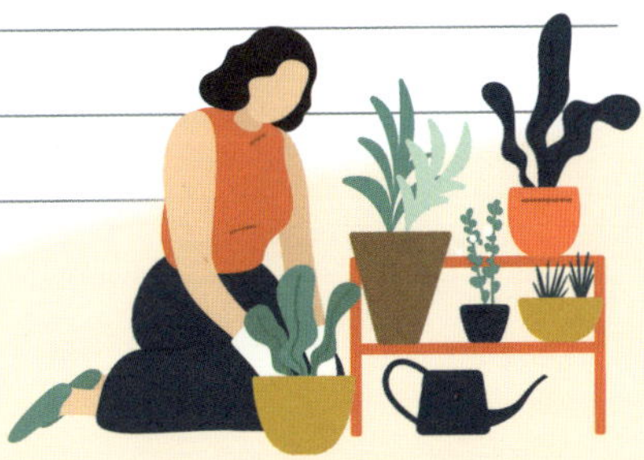

Do you draw people to you? At social events, do you seek out others and generate conversations, or do you hide in a corner, hoping no one talks to you? What are things you could do to feel more comfortable?

Do you reciprocate kindnesses? Do you tell acquaintances that you appreciate them? Do you do something to show your appreciation? How could you improve on these skills?

“We are not who other people say we are. We are who we know ourselves to be, and we are what we love. That’s okay.”

LAVERNE COX

CHAPTER 6

STRENGTHEN YOUR RELATIONSHIPS

It's not just the lack of social connection that results in loneliness. It's also the feeling that you don't have trustworthy, reciprocal, intimate friends with whom you can share the most salient details of your life. It's the lack of internal intimacy that leaves many of us feeling that we are alone in the world. Strengthening the personal relationships that you already have is essential to staving off internal loneliness and living a more productive, happy life. Let's discuss some relational skills that can bolster your ability to deepen your friendships.

LEARN HOW TO HANDLE CONFLICT

Conflict and disagreements are inevitable in human relationships. Two people can't possibly have the same needs, wants, opinions, and expectations at all times. When conflict is handled in an unhealthy manner, it can cause irreparable rifts, resentments, and break-ups. But when conflict is resolved in a healthy way, it increases your understanding of the other person, builds trust, and strengthens your relationships. When conflict isn't perceived as threatening or punishing, it fosters freedom, creativity, and safety in relationships. To better manage conflict, consider the following guidelines:

> "The single strongest predictor of thriving is good relationships with other people. It's not just emotional well-being and happiness—it's physical thriving. It's staying healthier and living longer."
>
> DR. ROBERT WALDINGER,
>
> *THE GOOD LIFE*

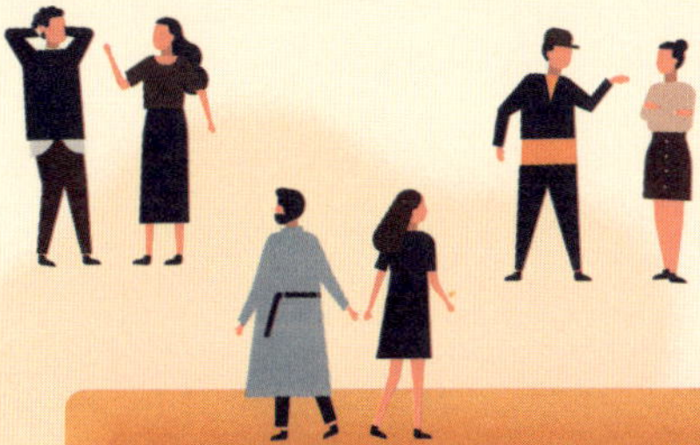

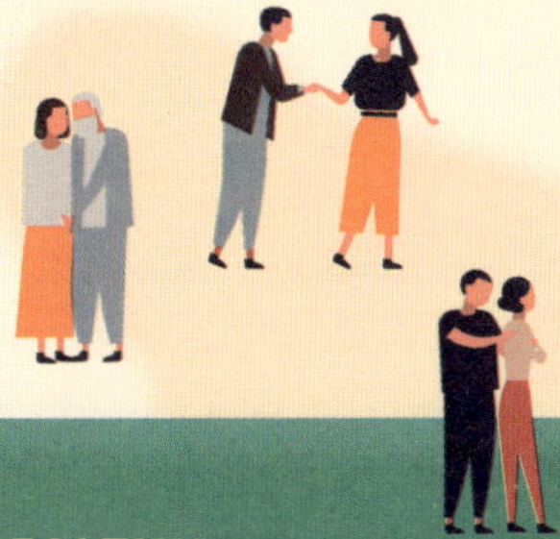

UNHEALTHY RESPONSES TO CONFLICT	HEALTHY RESPONSES TO CONFLICT
Inability to recognize and respond to what matters to the other person	Ability to empathize with the other person's point of view
Explosive, angry, hurtful, and resentful reactions	Calm, non-defensive, and respectful reactions
Withdrawal of love, resulting in rejection, isolation, shaming, and fear of abandonment	A readiness to forgive and forget and to move past conflict without holding resentments or anger
Inability to compromise or see the other person's side	Ability to seek compromise and avoid punishing
Feeling fearful or avoiding conflict; expecting a bad outcome	A belief that facing conflict head-on is best for both side

Do you often have conflicts in your relationships? Which ones are most worrisome?

What most often causes conflict? What's beneath the conflict?

How do you handle conflict when it arises? Is it working for you?

How can you address any conflicts and move forward in a more congenial way?

"If you are afraid of being lonely, don't try to be right."

JULES RENARD

DEEPEN CONVERSATIONS BY ASKING QUESTIONS

According to Kira Asatryan, author of *Stop Feeling Lonely*, to improve your ability to ask questions that foster intimacy, try the following: Pretend you are talking to your favorite character from a book or movie and desperately want to know a lot more about her. Then, based on what you already know about her, thoughtfully pose ten questions designed to elicit detailed information about her past or future specifically. This helps you learn how to deepen conversations and thereby foster greater intimacy in your relationships.

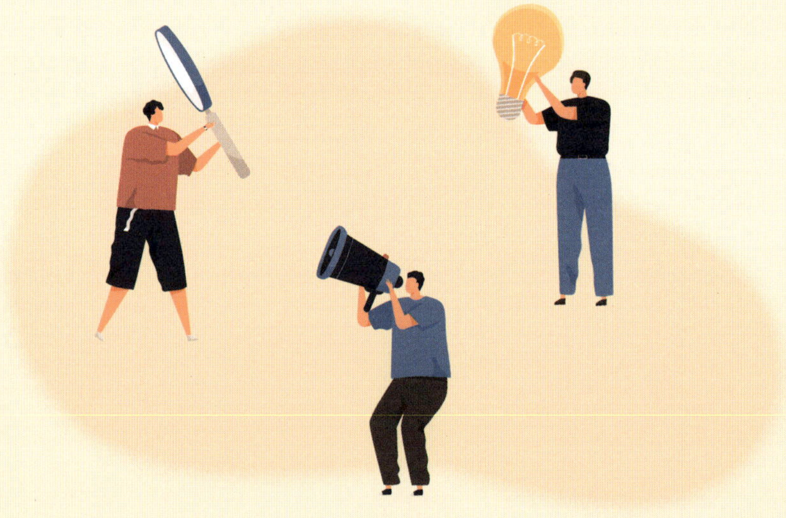

Imagine the character you want to know a lot more about and write a list of ten probing (but kind) questions that you would ask to discover a lot more about what makes them tick, what their fears are, what they want most in the world, what drives them, what they think is their best qualities, or where they feel lacking, and so on.

1

2

3

4

5

6

7

8

9

10

BE MORE SUPPORTIVE

It's important to offer emotional support to deepen relationships. Here are four ways you can be more supportive and thus draw your friends and family closer:

- **Emotional Social Support** is achieved by offering affirmations of someone's worth, expressing concern about someone's feelings, and sharing your positive regard for them. Simply listening to and validating feelings, letting others know they are valued, and being fully present when needed bolsters emotional support.
- **Informational Social Support** means sharing or receiving advice or information that can help someone who is experiencing a stressor or challenge they don't know how to handle. Listening closely, then gently suggesting experts who may offer advice, helpful books, local clinics, or groups, or sharing your experiences to suggest proactive solutions provides informational support.
- **Tangible Social Support** means doing kind and helpful favors to help others, such as providing financial support, offering to pay for their dinner, offering to share childcare duties, helping a friend move, or bringing a meal to someone sick or grieving. Doing helpful things for others fosters mutual trust, positive feelings, and a healthy interdependence.
- **Inclusive Social Support** is achieved by including friends in a group and spending time with friends who need support and may feel alone. This fosters a sense of *belonging* that strengthens bonds. By helping others feel more accepted, you create goodwill and a bond that will surely grow.

Which areas of support do you need to bolster?

How and with whom can you offer more emotional support?

How and with whom can you offer more informational support?

How and with whom can you offer more tangible support?

How and with whom can you offer more social support?

If you're not feeling supported in your relationships, what needs to change? Do you need new friends, or do you need to be more open and ask for support?

Do you let your friends know when *you* need support?

What kind of support do you need right now, and whom could you ask to provide it?

"The opposite of loneliness is not togetherness, it's intimacy.

RICHARD BACH

THREE WAYS TO CONNECT ON A DEEPER LEVEL

Dr. Marissa Franco suggests three ways to connect on a deeper level:

1. **Pick people on the same wavelength.** Choose people with qualities you want to develop—to be more fun-loving, to become more spiritual, to master an art, or to devote yourself to learning. Mutual interests make it easier for both of you to like each other and want more time together.

2. **Make yourself vulnerable.** Without burdening other people, instead of presenting what you imagine is a desirable persona, risk simply being yourself and being willing to share intimate details of your life. Research has shown that the more we intimately self-disclose, the more people like us.

3. **Show up when they need you.** Nothing bonds two people more than being there when the other truly needs emotional or physical support. If your new friend is going through a hard time, provide what they need, from childcare, meals delivered, their errands run, or someone to listen and genuinely care.

"Men who have a tempestuous inner life and do not seek to give vent to it by talking or writing are simply men who have no tempestuous inner life. Give company to a lonely man, and he will talk more than anyone."

CESARE PAVESE,

THIS BUSINESS OF LIVING

FOCUS ON KINDNESS

If you approach life with the intention to be kind to others, you will naturally treat others with the kind of respect that fosters connection. It's as simple as pausing when interacting to ask yourself:

- How might kindness improve this situation?
- How can I treat others with respect?
- How can I be of service to others?
- How can I show my concern for and commitment to others?

Kindness can be as simple as smiling and greeting those you pass on the street, holding the door for the person behind you, offering your space in line to an older woman, offering to help someone with their packages, or buying coffee for the stranger behind you in line. Being kind to others is guaranteed to make you feel better about yourself, and the more often that happens, the more you'll attract other people.

"Turn into the kind heart you are most looking for in another."

JOHN DE RUITER

When was the last time you were kind to a stranger? How often do you offer kindness to your friends? Your family? List five ways you can be kind on a regular basis.

TRY A LOVING-KINDNESS MEDITATION

Studies have shown that meditating for seven minutes, during which you purposely extend love and kindness to yourself and others, can help *you* feel more connected to others in a deep-seated way. To achieve this, sit comfortably, then take three or more slow, deep inhalations and complete exhalations. Let go of any concerns or mental preoccupations and simply focus on the breath moving down and back up through the center of your chest, in the area of your heart. Mentally repeat: *May I be happy. May I be well. May I be safe. May I be peaceful and at ease.* Then, think of someone you care about and send them loving-kindness by mentally repeating: *May Thomas be happy. May Thomas be well. May Thomas be safe. May Thomas be peaceful and at ease.* You can extend your loving-kindness to anyone and everyone, even—or especially to—people with whom you are frustrated or angry, as a means of release.

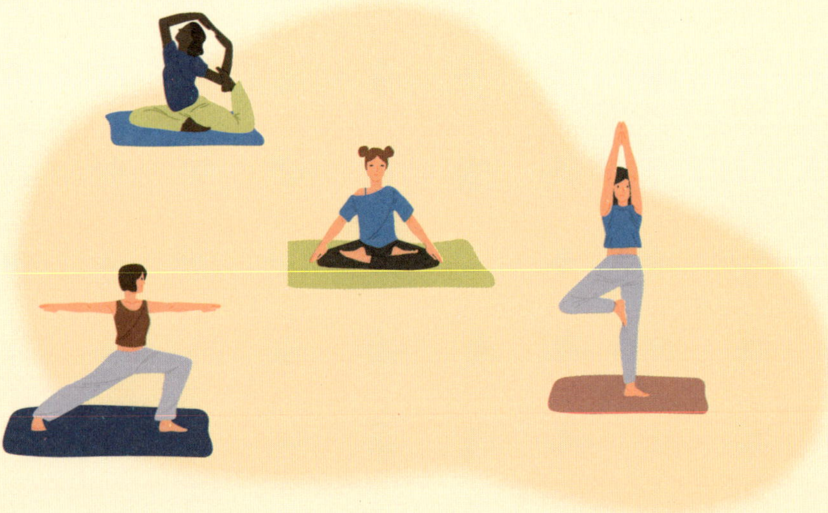

How did it feel to focus love and kindness toward yourself?

Were you able to take in the positive feelings and allow yourself to feel loved?

Who did you also send love and kindness to? Why them? Write down a few ways you could extend love and kindness to them and others in the coming days.

EMBRACE TIME SPENT ALONE

We often fear that we'll feel most lonely when alone, but solitude can be a reinvigorating time, particularly if you spend it doing something you love. You can blast your favorite music and dance around your living room, dive into a hobby you love, eat whatever appeals, binge-watch something only you want to see, or simply make choices that are entirely your own. Being alone is often the only time when a lack of stimulation or distractions inadvertently provides replenishment and even bliss. Beneath your thoughts and emotions lies a vast ocean of silence, peace, and well-being. The more you can access that space, the more that sense of well-being also permeates the rest of your day.

"When I was around eighteen,
I looked in the mirror and said,
'You're either going to love
yourself or hate yourself.'
And I decided to love myself.
That changed a lot of things."

QUEEN LATIFAH

List five things you could do when alone that you would thoroughly enjoy. It could be a hobby, a movie you want to watch, or a long, hot bath. Use the list to make any alone time true "me time."

> "There are some places in life where you can only go alone. Embrace the beauty of your solo journey."
>
> **MANDY HALE,**
>
> *THE SINGLE WOMAN: LIFE, LOVE, AND A DASH OF SASS*

FIND NEW HOBBIES

Spending your time on unfulfilling activities can contribute to unhappiness and boredom. These feelings may not directly cause loneliness, but they can certainly contribute to dissatisfaction with life, which can negatively affect how you feel about spending time with others. When you devote your free time to things you really enjoy, it's a form of self-respect. Hobbies are an important aspect of self-care that helps improve your outlook and give you more energy for meaningful connections. Hobbies also put you in touch with other people who enjoy similar activities, opening the door to more satisfying relationships. What hobbies could you pursue?

IMPROVE THE QUALITY OF RELATIONSHIPS

It's important to dive beneath surface pleasantries and bolster intimacy to deepen relationships. Being your authentic self and being vulnerable enough to share yourself are two ways to bolster intimacy. Other ways you can improve the quality of your current relationships are:

- When with others, go beyond surface dialogue and initiate a conversation about current events or other topics important to you. Ask for, pay attention to, and respect others' strong opinions and feelings.
- Call or visit loved ones. Face-to-face interaction always trumps digital interaction.
- Participate in activities current or potential friends love. Take up a sport they enjoy, go on a long hike together, volunteer together, or work on a project together. Togetherness will deepen your bond.
- Practice kindness. Surprise a friend with a bouquet or a book you know she'd love, return your neighbor's recycling containers to their storage area, or offer dinner to a friend who had a bad day.

How can you improve the quality of your most important relationships? What activities could you plan?

How can you show kindness to someone special?

"To be oneself, simply oneself, is so amazing and utterly unique an experience that it's hard to convince oneself so singular a thing happens to everybody."

SIMONE DE BEAUVOIR

TOUCH BASE MORE OFTEN

One simple way to deepen your existing relationships is to touch base more often. Rather than waiting for special occasions or preplanned events, regularly checking in with friends fosters intimacy. Not waiting for a reason to reach out and simply connecting to share the ordinariness of everyday life deepens the existing connection. When you do touch base, call rather than text, or better yet, Facetime or Zoom so you can see each other.

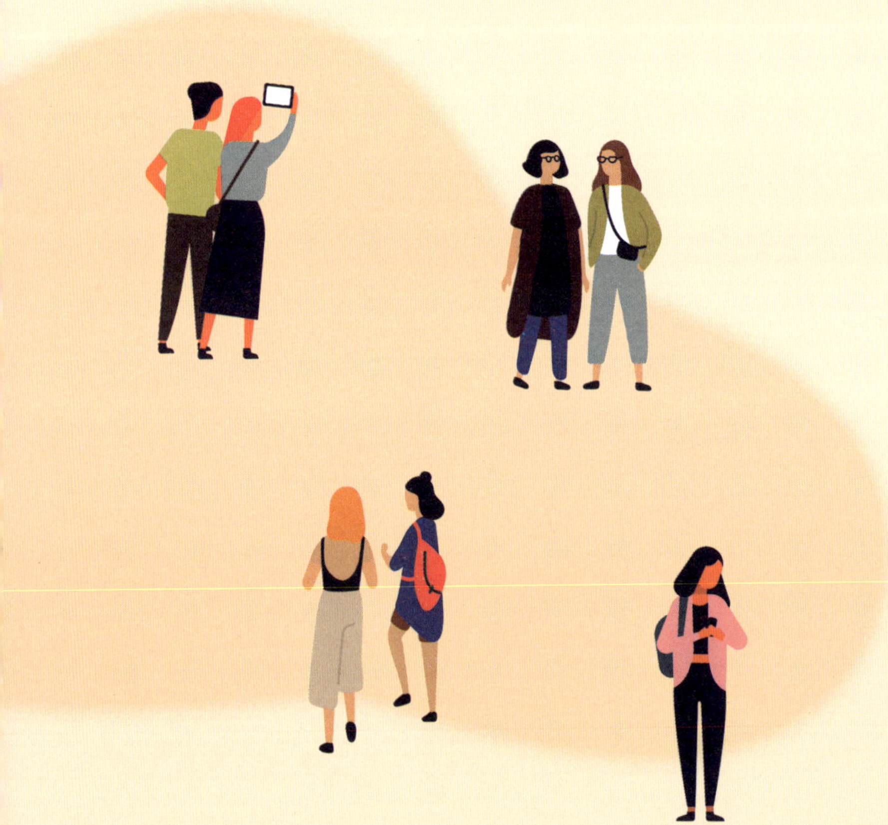

List three friends you could call on a more regular basis. Put reminders to touch base with them at least once a week in your calendar for the next three months or until it becomes a habit.

"A lesson of *Star Trek* (the Enterprise's crew)... may be that we find companionship not with our own, those like us, but with those others, unlike us, even aliens, with whom all we share is a voyage of loneliness."

PETER HO

CHAPTER 7

EXPAND YOUR SOCIAL CIRCLES

FIND COMMUNITY

For hundreds of years, belonging to a religious or faith-based group with shared values and beliefs provided regular social contact, communal support, meaning, and purpose. In 1999, 70 percent of Americans said they belonged to a church, synagogue, or mosque; by 2020, it had dropped to 47 percent, which means we're losing important pillars of community connection in our society. To feel less lonely, find a community of like-minded people and cultivate potential for deep friendships by:

- Seeking diverse friendships beyond your background and experiences
- Planning social events and inviting lots of new people
- Signing up for classes and talking to fellow participants
- Joining civic or community groups (fitness, religion, hobbies, professional, community) to foster a sense of belonging, meaning, and purpose and community
- Asking your local library for resources; they may offer book clubs you can conduct out of your home.

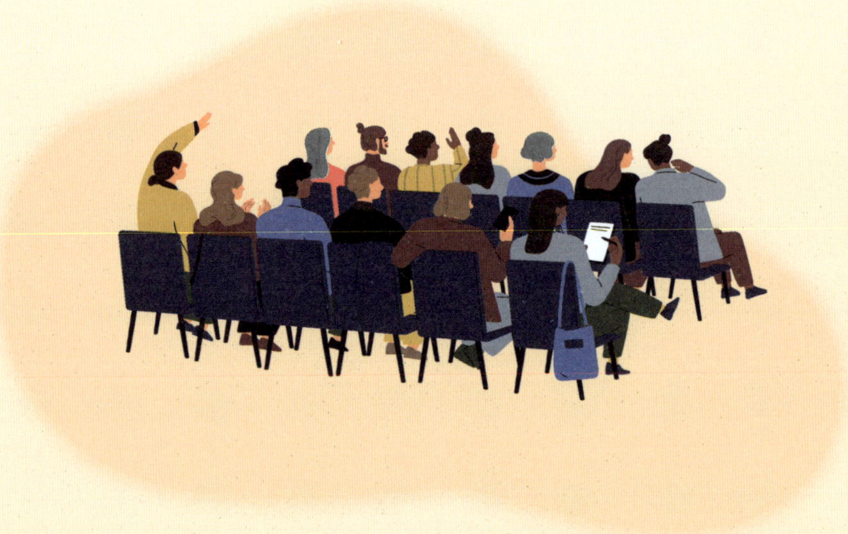

Which areas of your life seem ripe for expansion and finding people with whom you might discover a lot in common?

Where might you find people who have far different interests? Which ones are you willing to explore?

Research online to find three classes that you'd like to take and sign up for them!

What else could you do to expand your social circle?

FIND THE "WHY" IN DISCOMFORT

If you're someone who experiences social anxiety or simply is more introverted and less likely to force yourself to reach out, identifying the reason that you're making social expansion a goal will help you push past any resistance. Liz Moody, author of *100 Ways to Change Your Life*, said finding the "why" in establishing new habits is essential to creating and sticking to them. Instead of focusing on *how* you can push past your comfort level to seek and find new friends or deepen existing relationships, focus more on *why* you want to do this. Discovering "why" branching out is important to you—particularly when it syncs with your values and goals—will also bolster motivation. Perhaps you're reaching out to spread more kindness in the world or to be a faithful, helpful companion to others. Or maybe you want to help others find new friends and deepen their social connections. Whatever aligns with your deepest values can be a source of both inspiration and motivation.

Discovering "why" branching out is important to you—particularly when it syncs with your values and goals—will also bolster motivation. Perhaps you're reaching out to spread more kindness in the world or to be a faithful, helpful companion to others. Or maybe you want to help others find new friends and deepen their social connections. Whatever aligns with your deepest values can be a source of both inspiration and motivation.

Give thought as to why it's important for you to branch out, find new friends, and deepen current relationships. List all the positive reasons, particularly the ones that align with your values. Whenever you feel hesitant to reach out, review your list of "whys" and get yourself out there.

> “We tend to over-index slightly on the ‘how’ and under-index slightly on the ‘why.’”
>
> DANIEL PINK

BE OPEN-MINDED

When we meet someone new, we often make assumptions about someone’s personality, temperament, interests, intelligence, or values, but in doing so, we lose an opportunity to discover who they really are (which might turn out to be far more interesting or deep than we first imagined). Instead, avoid prejudgment, sit back, and patiently *allow* the new person to reveal (or create) who they are over time. This encourages both of you to remain open to learning more about each other and perhaps discovering surprising mutuality.

ATTRACT THE FRIENDS YOU WANT

Instead of allowing physical proximity to primarily determine who becomes a friend, consider seeking out the kind of people you want as friends. Do you want friends who challenge your thinking? Energize you and inspire you to new heights? Encourage you to be more charitable? Lure you far outside your cocoon? Coax you into pursuing your art? Devote themselves to doing good in the world? Volunteer to tutor underprivileged children? Go line dancing twice a week? Travel to foreign countries on adventures? Once you establish the kind of friends you seek, make a concerted effort to go where you can find them, and when you do, extend the hand of friendship.

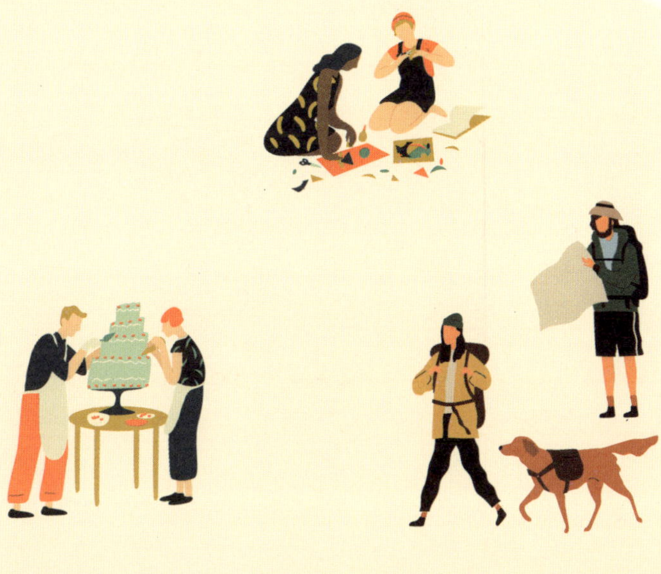

What kinds of friends do you want? List at least five possibilities and then explain *why* those particular characteristics are important to you. Do you already know people who fit? If you don't, where can you go to find the desired new acquaintances?

"I am lonely, yet not everybody will do. I don't know why some people fill the gaps, and others emphasize my loneliness."

ANAÏS NIN

> "When you're surrounded by all these people, it can be lonelier than when you're by yourself. You can be in a huge crowd, but if you don't feel like you can trust anyone or talk to anybody, you feel like you're really alone."
>
> FIONA APPLE

FIND YOUR TRIBE

Studies show that finding a community connection can be pivotal for mental wellness. Finding and hanging out with *like-minded* souls is a great way to combat loneliness *and* reinvigorate your passions. Whatever you love to do is an ideal place to start. Find classes or meetups, or simply go where you're most likely to find your tribe and use the opportunity to approach potential friends.

PURSUE FRIENDSHIPS

According to Dr. Marissa G. Franco, author of *Platonic: How the Science of Attachment Can Help You Make—and Keep—Friends*, the more we are simply exposed to others, the more we unconsciously accept and like them. Recurrence exposure fosters a bond. "They don't even have to say anything to us. It's completely unconscious," Dr. Franco said.

Thus, once you've met a potential friend, it's important to make recurring plans to see them. Increasing exposure over time makes it more likely that you'll form a lasting relationship. That said, it's also important that you proceed slowly, allowing both of you to establish trust and intimacy at each person's pace. Start by hanging out together, meeting for dinner, going to a movie, visiting an art museum, or other activities that will be fun for you both. Over time, slowly reveal more of yourself and encourage them to reciprocate. Then, keep making future plans to be together.

Is there anyone in your life that you'd like to see more? List three activities you could do with them, invite them to join you, and put the dates in your calendar.

CHOOSE YOUR FRIENDS WISELY

Seeking new friends doesn't mean gathering people indiscriminately and latching onto them. While it's wise to expand the type of people you usually befriend, it's also wise to assess whether they're true friend material. If you're not sure, ask yourself:

- Does our conversation flow easily, or does it feel forced?
- Do they seem to understand, accept, and support you truly?
- Do you truly understand, accept, and support them?
- Do you feel better or worse about yourself when you're with them?
- Do you feel energized or depleted after being with them?
- Do you include them in your life for the positive qualities they have or just to have more people in your life?

While being with someone (anyone) may help you feel less lonely at the moment, select people with the most potential for long-lasting friendships, and you'll definitely feel less lonely down the line.

Friendships can naturally evolve, sometimes growing stronger and other times falling apart. Have you ever experienced a friendship breakup? Was it a slow fade as your lives drifted in different directions or a more abrupt end? What did you learn from the experience?

BE A FUN MAGNET

According to Cathrine Price, author of *The Power of Fun*, being upbeat, positive, and fun attracts people and keeps them coming back. She has a five-prong approach to being a fun magnet:

1. **Stay open to new ideas.** Negativity turns off people. Even if what they say sounds crazy, avoid dismissing their ideas. Stay open to discussing them further and looking for ways to build on them.

2. **Don't put yourself down.** Instead of pointing out and apologizing for your shortcomings, learn to see your foibles as an indication that you're human, and better yet, learn to laugh at yourself.

3. **Surrender center stage.** When you barrage others with humor or stories designed to put yourself center stage, it shuts down conversation. Instead, focus on the other person and be their receptive, reactive audience.

4. **Draw them out.** The more you're drawing someone out by asking questions, being upbeat, and laughing along with them, the more they'll want to see you again.

5. **Give them your full attention.** These days, in particular, turning off your phone, looking directly into someone's eyes, listening closely to what they're saying, and appropriately responding fosters intimacy. It is far more likely to create the kind of deeper connection you crave.

This doesn't mean you cannot occasionally be sad or vulnerable. As relationships deepen, being vulnerable fosters intimacy, but in the beginning stages of forming friendships, it's better to present your more upbeat self. Meditate before you go out, focusing on all the positives in your life, then go out and share them.

"The vast majority of us are in the same boat—wanting to connect, wanting to talk about something *real* that lets us think and feel seen and heard, but getting to that place isn't always easy or natural."

LIZ MOODY

BECOME A GOOD CONVERSATIONALIST

Instead of striving so hard to appear interesting when talking with others, it's far more important to be a good listener, someone who pays attention while others talk and then asks questions related to what they revealed. According to dating expert Logan Ury, the key to being liked by people is to be *interested* rather than *interesting*. "Research shows that asking people questions that make them feel interesting is what makes *them* attracted to you. The more the other person talks, the more they think you're a great conversationalist."

Four ways to be a better conversationalist are:

HAVE SOMETHING TO TALK ABOUT

Stay current on a wide range of topics and use whatever recently caught your interest to initiate and expand conversations. Be prepared to share your thoughts and then focus on encouraging the other person to share their thoughts.

ASK QUESTIONS

When someone expresses interest in something, take the opportunity to ask them questions that will expand the conversation. Don't deflect or share a similar experience. Instead, ask more about their experience.

LISTEN PROACTIVELY

Instead of thinking ahead to what you might say next, pay close attention to what the other person is saying and respond to what they said rather than what you might have thought. Encourage them to talk more about their thoughts, feelings, and interests.

NOTICE WHAT LIGHTS THEM UP

We can all tell when a topic excites someone. Take notice and use their excitement to spark additional conversation by asking questions related to what created the spark.

Remember, the more you focus on the other person and encourage them to shine, the more they'll like talking with you. As the relationship deepens, the conversation will become more reciprocal and offer opportunities for you to share more about yourself.

List five topics that you know a lot about and can offer scintillating conversation on when needed.

1

2

3

4

5

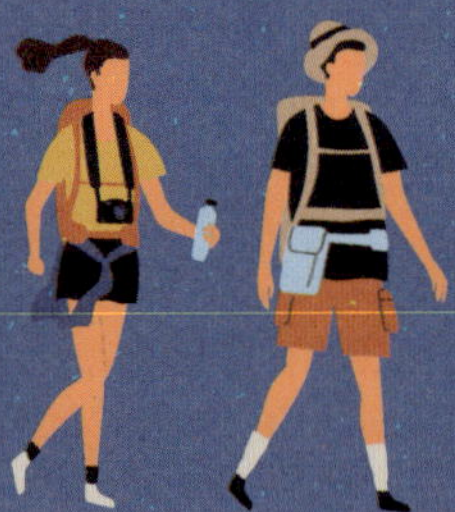

List five things that have always fascinated you and then learn more about them so you'll have more to talk about in social settings.

1

2

3

4

5

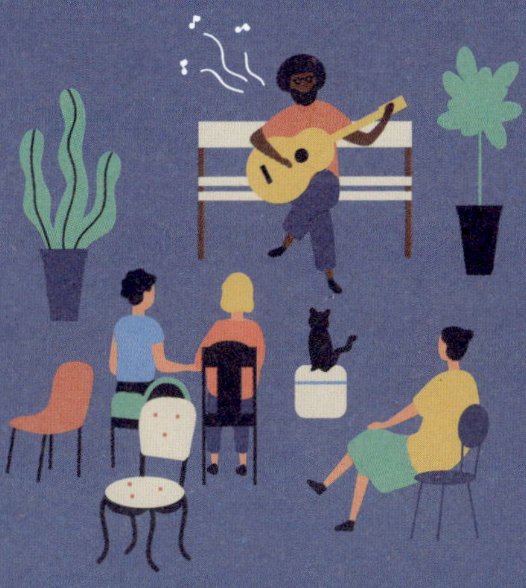

FIND A CAUSE THAT INSPIRES YOU

It's not only a surefire way to meet kind-hearted people, but it will help you view yourself as a generous, thoughtful, giving person and thereby bolster your self-esteem. According to Mike Rucker, PhD, author of *The Fun Habit, How the Pursuit of Joy and Wonder Can Change Your Life*, being thoughtful about how you direct your community engagement will help you fulfill the three basic psychological needs: autonomy, competence, and relatedness. He suggests you:

1. **Pick a cause that's personal.** When it's personal and uniquely meaningful, volunteering expands your sense of autonomy. Choose something that matters, and it will also boost motivation and self-esteem.

2. **Use your personality and skill set.** Making the best use of your personality and exercising your unique skills in service to others boosts your feeling of competence, which may also improve your work performance or level of ambition.

3. **Share your enthusiasm with others.** When you're authentically volunteering and sharing your enthusiasm with others, it helps you to relish the experience, deepen your commitment, and enhance your sense of relatedness.

When you're offering your services from intrinsic compassion and a genuine desire to be of service, it creates motivation that lasts—and decreases the likelihood that you'll be lonely.

"Help one person at a time, and always start with the person nearest you."

MOTHER THERESA

List at least five causes or charities that are personal to you. If you can't think of any, go online to research possibilities.

1

2

3

4

5

List five aspects of your personality and your skills that you could offer.

1

2

3

4

5

Name five people you would share your enthusiasm about this new pursuit with.

1

2

3

4

5

"We are social animals. Like all social animals, a person who is selfish will not attract others, but a person who helps others will invite the kindness and company of others."

TODD PERELMUTER

Places to look for volunteering opportunities include:

- **Church Organizations.** Most churches have multiple volunteer opportunities. Even if you're not a member, they'd likely welcome your help.

- **Local charities.** Your local Chamber of Commerce likely has a list of local charities looking for volunteers.

- **Food banks.** These organizations always need help.

- **Tutoring opportunities.** Contact local schools or search for educational associations. Often, you'll find opportunities to either teach skills or simply to spend time with students, reading or relating to them.

Use online resources to find volunteer opportunities. Often, there's a local association or online "newspaper" that lists all volunteer opportunities in your community.

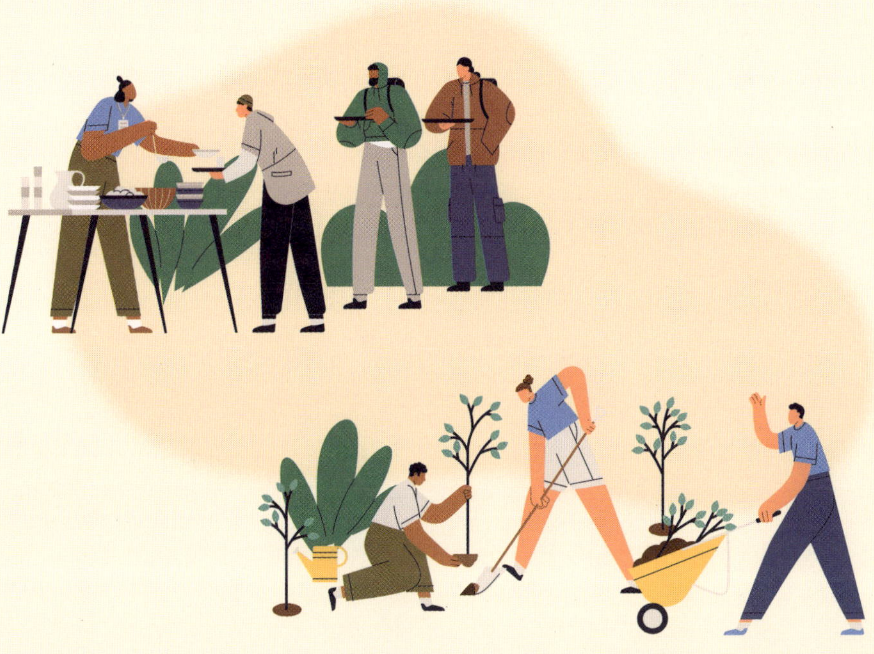

List five possibilities for volunteering, then pick at least one to dip your toes in the water.

1

2

3

4

5

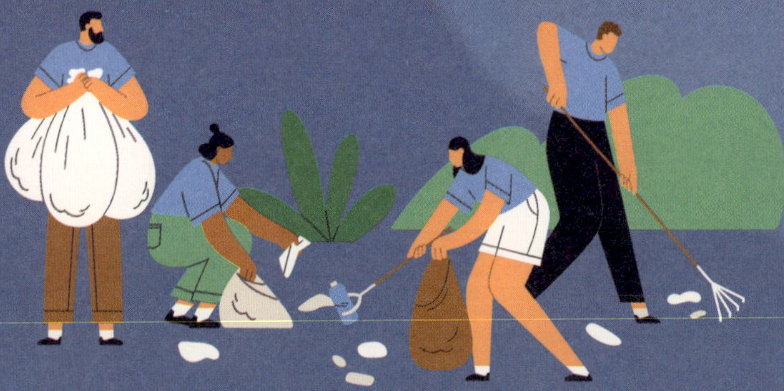

"Spirituality is recognizing and celebrating that we are all inextricably connected to each other by a power greater than all of us, and that our connection to the power and to one another is grounded in love and compassion."

BRENÉ BROWN

GET PHYSICAL

Simply moving your body not only improves your health but also improves your mood and perhaps gets you out and about, meeting other people. Sign up for dance classes, yoga, or other forms of exercise that require leaving your house. Try joining a sports club, like pickleball or tennis. Go hiking or bird watching with others (you can find groups online). Check for local walking tours or charity runs. If all else fails, go for a walk alone (while enjoying nature). Staying active eases depression, anxiety, stress, and a host of other things that can come with feeling lonely.

ADOPT A DOG

Rescuing a pet can help alleviate loneliness by combining the benefits of altruism and companionship. You feel good about providing a needed home. The pet offers companionship and reciprocal, unconditional affection. Plus, walking a dog opens you up to a community of other dog-walkers, as a cute dog on a leash tends to be a people magnet. As a bonus, research suggests having a pet can lower blood pressure, improve your mood, and ease stress. If you're not able to adopt a pet, perhaps foster puppies, volunteer to work at your local pet shelter, or look for dog-walking opportunities as a way to maximize your time with animals *and* give back to the community.

List five activities you enjoy and choose three to do in the coming weeks.

1

2

3

4

5

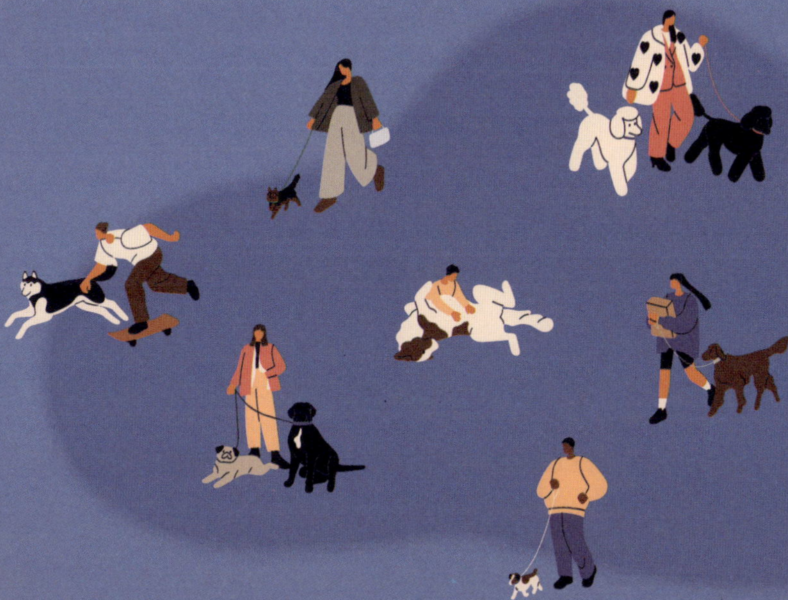

"If you don't risk anything,
you risk even more.

ERICA JONG

CHAPTER 8

SEEK HELP WHEN STRUGGLING

TAKE THE FIRST STEPS

To overcome loneliness, simply start by recognizing that you are lonely and that loneliness is not something shameful but merely a sign that you both need and crave social connection. As we've discussed throughout this book, you can take specific, numerous steps to ease loneliness. While your life won't dramatically change overnight, taking those first steps toward bolstering your self-esteem, strengthening your social skills, reaching out, deepening relationships, and expanding your social circle will help relieve your feelings of loneliness and build connections that support your well-being.

If you've worked your way through this book and still feel lonely, you can likely find a host of resources online, from support groups to meetup opportunities. Even Facebook facilitates local groups where people can meet to enjoy shared activities. Keep bravely putting yourself out there. Trust that there are people out there waiting to connect with you who are just as scared to make the first move.

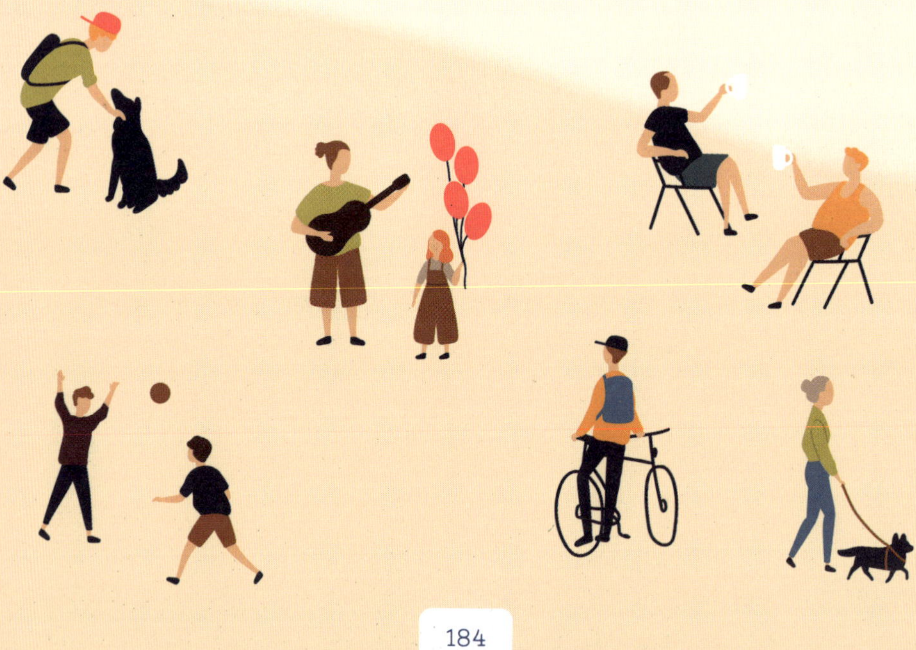

If you continue to struggle, perhaps it's time to reach out to someone. Start by confiding in someone you know loves and supports you, someone you trust with your deepest feelings. Often, we are afraid that revealing our vulnerabilities will make us appear weak but opening up is an act of courage. Being honest and vulnerable can help create the kind of connection you crave.

If you need additional support, talk to your minister or doctor, who'll likely recommend a social worker or counselor. Even short-term therapy can be helpful in breaking down barriers, and online therapy can be a great option because it allows you to contact a therapist whenever it is convenient for you. Rather than resist that step, avail yourself of any opportunities to discuss your feelings, your fears, and any roadblocks you've encountered to forming new friendships. Perhaps all you need is someone to support your efforts, cheer you on, and help you feel more comfortable with yourself and the process. They can also help you better understand yourself and boost your self-esteem, both of which will improve your ability to form social connections.

Remember that everyone seeks social connection, and people need you as much as you need them.

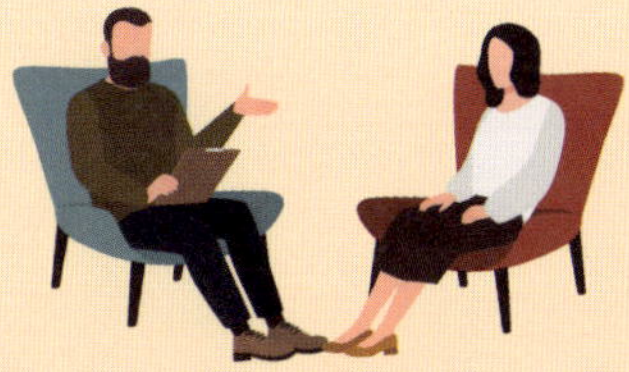

Who is someone you can reach out to? What can you share with them?

What are your fears about being vulnerable and sharing your struggles?

Reflect on your feelings now versus when you started this workbook. Have you made any progress?

Have you made any new friends or deepened your relationship with others?

WHERE TO FIND HELP

The Substance Abuse and Mental Health Services Administration (SAMHSA) will help you locate mental health treatment facilities and programs. To find a facility in your state, search SAMHSA's online Behavioral Health Treatment Services Locator . For additional resources, visit the National Institute of Mental Health NIMH's Help for Mental Illnesses web page.

"Above all, be the heroine of your life, not the victim."

NORA EPHRON

RESOURCES

Anderson, G. and Nadel, J. (2017). *We: A Manifesto for Women Everywhere.* United States: Atria Books.

Asatryan, K. (2016). *Stop Being Lonely: Three Simple Steps to Developing Close Friendships.* United States: New World Library.

Bass, D. (2018). *Grateful: The Transformative Power.* United States: Harper One.

Beck, M. (2021). *The Way of Integrity : Finding the Path to Your True Self.* United States: The Open Field.

Brach, T. (2020). *Radical Compassion: Learning to Love Yourself and Your World.* United States: Penguin Life.

Brown, B. (2014). *Braving the Wilderness: The Quest for True Belonging and the Courage.* United States: Random House.

Cherry, K. and Mattiuzzi, P. (2010). *Everything Psychology: Explore The Human Psyche and Understand Why We Do The Things We Do.* United States: Adams Media.

Dembling, S. (2015). *Introverts in Love: The Quiet Way to Happily Ever After.* United States: TarcherPerigee.

Elliot, E. (2007). *The Path of Loneliness.* United States: Revell.

Franco, M., PhD (2022). *Platonic: How the Science of Attachment Can Help You Make—and Keep—Friends.* United States: G.P. Putnam.

Garret, N. (2022). *The Lonely Stories: 22 Celebrated Writers on the Joys & Struggles of Being Alone.* United States: Catapult.

Gordon, M. 12 Ways to Beat Loneliness. webmd.com.

Han, S. (2021). You Can Only Maintain So Many Close Friendships. *Atlantic Monthly.*

Hunt, MG, Marx, R, Lipson, C, and Young, J (2018). No More FOMO: Limiting Social Media Decreases Loneliness and Depression. *Journal of Social and Clinical Psychology.*

Kabat-Zinn, J. (2017). *Wherever You Go, There You Are: Mindfulness Meditation in Everyday Life.* United States: Hachette Books.

Moody, L. (2023). *100 Ways to Change Your Life: The Science of Leveling Up Health, Happiness, Relationships & Success.* United States: Harper Wave.

Murther, V. M.D., Surgeon General of the United States *(2023). Together: The Healing Power of Human Connection in a Sometimes Lonely World.* United States: Harper Paperbacks.

Office of the Surgeon General. (2023). *Our Epidemic of Loneliness and Isolation: The US Surgeon General's Advisory on the Healing Effects of Social Connection and Community.* U.S. Department of Health and Human Services, Public Health Service, Office of the Surgeon General.

Paquette, J. (2020) *Awestruck: How Embracing Wonder Can Make You Happier, Healthier, and More Connected.* United States: Shambhala.

Price, C. (2024). *The Power of Fun: How to Feel Alive Again.* United States: Dial Press.

Rucker, M., PhD. (2023). *The Fun Habit: How the Pursuit of Joy and Wonder Can Change Your Life.* United States: Atria Books.

Salter Ainsworth, M. (2015). *Patterns of Attachment. United States:* Routledge.

Shetty, J. (2020). *Think Like a Monk: Train Your Mind for Peace and Purpose Every Day.* United States: Simon & Schuster.

Thaler, L.T., Koval, R., et al., (2018). *Grit To Great: How Perseverance, Passion, And Pluck Take You from Ordinary to Extraordinary.* United States: Currency.

Thomée, S. (2014). "Mobile Phone Use and Mental Health. A Review of the Research That Takes a Psychological Perspective on Exposure," *National Library of Medicine.*

Ury, L. (2021). *How to Not Die Alone: The Surprising Science That Will Help You Find Love.* United States: Simon & Schuster.

(2016). New Report Finds Teens Feel Addicted to Their Phones, Causing Tension at Home, *Common Sense Media.*

Websites

Elizabeth Scott PhD, *verywellmind.com.*

National Institute of Mental Health: nih.gov

Mentalhealthfoundation.org